Immunology for the Practicing Physician

Immunology for the Practicing Physician

Edited by
Jon R. Schmidtke and Ronald M. Ferguson

Departments of Surgery and Microbiology
University of Minnesota Medical School
Minneapolis, Minnesota

Plenum Press · New York and London

Library of Congress Cataloging in Publication Data

Main entry under title:

Immunology for the practicing physician.

"Proceedings of the Metropolitan Medical Center Symposium held in Minneapolis, Minnesota, April 30-May 1, 1976."
Includes index.
1. Immunologic diseases—Congresses. 2. Immunology—Congresses. I. Schmidtke, Jon R. II. Ferguson, Ronald M. III. Metropolitan Medical Center.
RC581.2.I45 616.07'9 77-2170
ISBN-13: 978-1-4615-8812-2 e-ISBN-13: 978-1-4615-8810-8
DOI: 10.1007/978-1-4615-8810-8

Proceedings of the Metropolitan Medical Center Symposium held in Minneapolis, Minnesota, April 30-May 1, 1976

Softcover reprint of the hardcover 1st edition 1977
A Division of Plenum Publishing Corporation
227 West 17th Street, New York, N.Y. 10011

Preface

The field of immunology has grown extensively during the past decade. The basic concepts and importance of these findings may have clinical application in the management, detection, and explanation of human diseases. Therefore, when a topic was to be chosen for the dedication of the new Metropolitan Medical Center, in Minneapolis, Minnesota, Immunology, and its relation to medicine, was selected. In fact, "applied immunology has had great impact on all aspects of medical practice. This impact has taken several forms: modern immunology has defined areas of new medical practice (in the immunodeficiency disease, for example); has lent strength to the development of other areas (such as transplantation and tumor immunology); has provided understanding of the etiology and pathogenesis of certain diseases; has provided investigative approaches in laboratory methods for the study of diseases; and may play a major role in diagnosis of treatment and cancer" (Lancet, April 19, 1976).

The purpose of this symposium was to bring to the practicing physician the current "state of the art" of immunological research in an interesting and comprehensible manner. It was our hope that practicing physicians would be updated regarding new aspects of basic and clinical concepts of cellular immunology. The symposium goal was to present clear discussions of the factors related to lymphocyte function in the expression of the immune response, both in normal and disease states. In the first half of this volume the basic fundamentals of cellular immunology are presented. Based on these concepts, the second half of the symposium was dedicated to the possible clinical relevance of basic immunology which currently faces practicing physicians.

As succinctly stated in the seminar brochure by Dr. Richard Reese, pathologist at Metropolitan Medical Center and Editor in

Chief of Minnesota Medicine; "immunology is where medicine's fundamental issues - the basic understanding of disease; its diagnosis, cause, and cure - will be decided. For it is the immune system that dictates how we react to or resist disease. This symposium featuring perhaps the finest collection of experts, will clarify for the practicing physician where we stand on these issues."

In the introduction the basic terminology of cellular immunology is presented by Dr. Jon R. Schmidtke. A discussion of lymphocyte cell surface receptors by Dr. Emil Unanue follows. Dr. David Katz presents the relationship between genes, cells and molecules of the immune response. The cellular regulation of the immune response is explained by Dr. Richard Gershon.

Armed with this basic knowledge of cellular immunology, Dr. Charles Cochrane presents a review of immune complex diseases and possible mechanisms and sites of manipulation for these diseases. Dr. Frank J. Dixon discusses current concepts of the role of chronic viral infection in immunologic diseases. Clinical renal allograft transplantation is approached by Dr. John S. Najarian. In renal allograft transplantation suppression of the immune response is the obvious goal. However, Dr. Richard L. Simmons explains current concepts of tumor immunotherapy in which it is desirable to augment the immune response. The relationship between the immune response and the capacity of the normal host to reject spontaneously arising tumors is discussed by Dr. Robert L. Schwartz and Dr. John Kersey.

We would like to take this opportunity to thank the staff of the Metropolitan Medical Center for making this symposium possible. Dr. John H. Linner, Chairman of the Seminar Committee, provided the impetus for the symposium. We would especially like to thank Ms. Rita Schiavino for her enduring efforts to bring about the mechanical aspects of this symposium. In addition, we would like to thank Ms. Nancy Nordhaugen and Ms. Carol Radermacher for expert typing assistance and assembling the manuscripts for this publication.

Jon R. Schmidtke, Ph.D.
Associate Professor
Surgery and Microbiology
University of Minnesota

Ronald M. Ferguson, M.D.
Medical Fellow
Department of Surgery
University of Minnesota

Contents

CURRENT CONCEPTS IN IMMUNOLOGY

Jon R. Schmidtke, Ph.D.

Departments of Surgery and Microbiology

University of Minnesota, Mpls., Mn 55455

Immunology is one of the most rapidly developing fields of medicine, and there are several questions basic to our understanding of it that we must answer before a thorough discussion can begin. 1) What series of cellular events take place in the host between the introduction of antigen and the synthesis of antibody? For example, when an injection of tetanus toxoid is given, what cells take up the toxoid and present the antigen to lymphocytes, and how do these lymphocytes interact to eventually synthesize anti-toxoid antibody? Furthermore, what cells are responsible for maintaining the "memory" so important for the tetanus toxoid boosters, or infection with the organism? 2) What cells and regulatory factors are involved between the time of implantation of an allograft or the development of a tumor, and subsequent rejection of the allograft and hopefully the rejection of the tumor? 3) How do the cells involved in the immune response develop embryologically and where are they found in the human lymphoid apparatus? 4) Do the cells involved in immune response possess any unique characteristics that make their identification, function, and quantitation possible for study or clinical evaluation, or both, in various disease states?

The obvious goal in understanding these processes is effective clinical manipulation and engineering of the immune response. We could therefore selectively augment the immune response, as in the case of a cell-mediated response to a tumor, or suppress the response in the case of a transplanted organ. Also, immunodiagnostic tests can be useful clinical reflections of the in vivo immune state.

Our immune system can be divided into three, time and functionally dependent areas (Figure 1). First, the afferent phase represents the factors and events that take place when an antigen, like tetanus toxoid or a foreign allograft, enters the host. Second, the central phase of the immune response can be divided into the functions of two broad categories of lymphocytes: the thymus derived (T) cell and the bone marrow derived (B) cell, and the macrophages. After injection, antigen is encountered first by macrophages, then by T cells and B cells. When the antigen is a soluble or particulate protein antigen, circulatory antibody is usually produced. The antibody can then react with either the original antigen, as in the case of tetanus toxoid, or the toxin from the bacteria if the host is infected. Thirdly, in the case of T cell-mediated immune responses to the implantation of an allograft or tumor, sensitized lymphocytes are produced which can act on the original immunizing allograft or tumor, if it is present. This last set of cellular events is called the efferent or effector phase of the immune response. We therefore have a) an afferent phase of the immune response, which is the introduction of the stimulus, b) the central phase of the immune response, with which most of this volume will deal, and c) the efferent or final phase of the immune response.

Figure I

Physiology of the Immune System

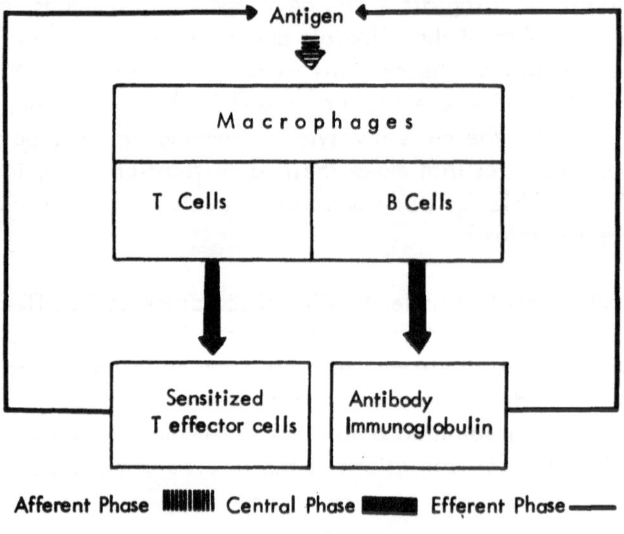

Before we can examine why lymphocytes are subdivided into T and B cells and how they function in the immune response, we need an experimental model. X-irradiated mice are deprived of their functional lymphoid tissue. When various lymphoid cell populations from gentically identical mice are selectively introduced into these x-rayed mice, cells will not be rejected. If a lethally x-irradiated (900r) mouse is not given any lymphoid cells before receiving a tetanus toxoid injection, the mouse produces no antibody before the animal dies (Table I). X-irradiation depletes the lymphoid apparatus which is therefore not able to respond to an antigenic stimulus and form antibodies. If we selectively introduce antigen and thymus cells into these x-rayed animals, a meager immune response takes place. In other words, T cells alone cannot reconstitute an x-irradiated mouse's ability to mount a significant antibody response. If we do the converse experiment and inject antigen and B cells, we again see only a meager antibody response. If, however, we inject antigen and both T and B cells, we see a significant, synergistic effect on the antibody response which is greater than the response made when animals received either T or B cell populations. We can conclude that T and B cells collaborate synergistically in the production of antibody to an antigen. T cells function as helper cells. After antigen contact, T cells either allow or induce B cells to undergo differentiation and proliferation into actual antibody secreting plasma cells. For animals to make an immune response to most antigens, the collaboration of T and B cells is needed. In Chapter 2, Dr. Unanue focuses on the interaction of antigens with the lymphocytes involved in the immune response. Dr. Katz describes in Chapter 3, how T and B cells interact and the genetic restrictions of their interaction. The regulatory or suppressor role that T cells can play in both enhancing and suppressing the immune response is discussed in Chapter 4 by Dr. Gershon.

Another broad category of the immune response is called cell mediated immunity. Cell mediated immune reactions are the exclusive property of the thymus derived, T cells. T cells acting alone can act as effector cells in the rejection of an allograft or tumor, and subpopulations of T cells can regulate the development and maturation of cell mediated immune reactions. T cells can actually destroy cells of allograft or tumor cells. Cell mediated immune reactions are characteristically called delayed type hypersensitivity. The PPD-

Table I

Synergistic collaboration in mice between thymus and bone marrow cells in the production of antibody to tetanus toxoid.

Mice (900r) plus:	Lymphoid Cells	Antibody
--	--	0
tetanus toxoid	bone marrow	10
tetanus toxoid	thymus	10
tetanus toxoid	bone marrow and thymus	90

Mice after irradiation are given nothing or antigen and lymphoid cells from normal, unirradiated, syngeneic mice. Antibody is assayed 5 days later. Data are presented as percent of control, unirradiated mice given tetanus toxoid alone.

tuberculin skin test is a classic example. Cell mediated immunity is involved in the resistance to intracellular infectious agents such as Listeria, Mycobacteria sp., protozoan parasites and many viruses. Graft-versus-host disease, as the result of bone marrow transplantation and immunodeficiency disease, are manifestations of cell mediated immune reactions, as are drug allergies and contact dermatitis. In Chapter 9, Dr. Kersey discusses specific defects that can be manifested in both the thymus and in bone marrow derived populations.

T and B lymphocytes collaborate, in an unknown way, to allow antibody production by B cells which have differentiated into plasma cells. In this system T cells act as regulator cells to both help and suppress antibody production. Cell mediated immune reactions are chiefly the response of T cells which effect the destruction of an allograft or tumor. Thymus derived cells can also amplify and suppress cell mediated immune reactions.

How do these independent lines of lymphocytes develop embryologically, where do they mature into immunocompetent cells that can recognize an antigen, and where are they located in the human body? The bone marrow contains a population of multipotential stem cells (Figure 2). These cells are undifferentiated in that they are not capable of specifically recognizing antigens. One line of stem cells, destined to become B lymphocytes, migrates or egresses from the bone marrow and matures into immunocompetent, antigen recognizing B cells in an unknown mammalian organ. In birds, this organ is the Bursa of Fabricius. After a period of maturation in this primary lymphoid organ, the B cells migrate and seed secondary lymphoid organs, such as lymph nodes, the appendix, gut associated lymphoid tissue, and the spleen. These cells have matured when they are capable of recognizing and responding to specific antigenic stimuli.

T cells develop independently from another precursor and mature in the thymus, which is the other primary lymphoid organ. Thymus cells then leave the thymus and also seed secondary lymphoid organs: the spleen, lymph nodes, and gut associated lymphoid tissue. The secondary lymphoid organs consist primarily of mixtures of T and B cells.

Figure 2

Ontogeny of Immunocompetent Cells

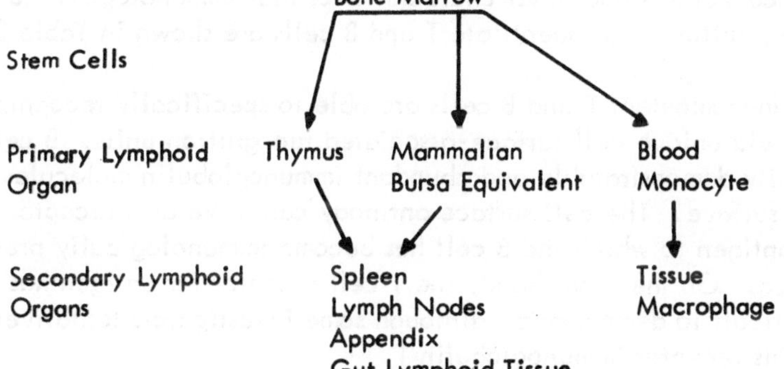

Lymphocyte multiplication and division in primary lymphoid organs is antigen independent while lymphocyte multiplication in secondary lymphoid organs is antigen dependent. In germ free animals the primary lymphoid organs are essentially the same size as those in conventional animals. However, the secondary lymphoid organs are markedly smaller in size in germ free animals. Upon antigenic stimulation lymphoid organs increase in size, as in "swollen lymph nodes". Macrophages have an essential regulatory role in the immune response and are also derived from bone marrow stem cell precursors. The bone marrow derived blood monocytes can be considered to be an immature macrophage. Upon migration into tissue, monocytes acquire the characteristics of tissue macrophages. These cells have a relatively non-specific, although essential, role in presenting antigens to immunocompetent T and B cells.

Histologically, T and B lymphocytes are found in defined areas of secondary lymphoid organs. In lymph nodes, the B cells are located in the primary follicles and germinal centers while T cells can be found in the paracortical regions. In the spleen, T lymphocytes are characteristically found in the periarteriolar region and the B cells are located in the germinal centers.

We have indicated that thymus derived and bone marrow derived cells have specific functions in the immune response. The next question is how do immunologists investigate these roles in the immune response? T and B cells have unique functional properties and cell surface markers so that these cells can be quantitatively and functionally assayed in both in vitro and in vivo immune systems. Some of the surface markers and other characteristics that immunologists use to define, follow, and quantitate T and B cells are shown in Table 2.

Immunocompetent T and B cells are able to specifically recognize antigens via unique cell surface-associated recognition units. B cells have easily demonstratable and abundant immunoglobulin molecules on their surface. The cell surface antibody can serve as a receptor for the antigen to which the B cell has become immunologically precommitted. On the other hand, the T cell receptor for antigen has been difficult to demonstrate, although some investigators tentatively called this receptor immunoglobulin T.

Table 2

Quantitative and Functional Characteristics of Murine T and B Cells

Characteristics	T cells	B cells
A. Cell Surface Antigens		
Θ	+	-
TL	+	-
Ly	+	-
H-2	+	+
Surface immunoglobulin*	-	+
PC	-	+ plasma cell
MBLA	-	+
B. Functional Analysis		
1. Mitogenic stimulation by:		
Phytohemagglutinin	+	-
Concanavalin A	+	-
Lipopolysaccharide	-	+
2. Role in antibody formation		
secretion of antibody	-	+
helper function	+	-
C. Inactivation by therapeutic agents		
x-irradiation	+	+++
antilymphocyte serum	+	+++
steroids	+	+

* easily demonstrable with present techniques

T and B cells also have other unique cell surface structures (antigens) which can be useful in quantitating mixed populations. These cell surface antigens are immunogenic. If we inject purified T cells bearing a unique marker into a mouse which lacks only this particular cell surface antigen the recipient mouse will make antibody to this unique cell surface antigen. Since this antibody will only react with cells bearing this antigen, we can use the antibody to quantitate and/or follow these cells. The θ or Thy 1.2 antigen is found only on the surface of T cells. Anti θ serum therefore will react specifically with T cells. The thymus leukemia (TL) antigen is found only on the thymus cells and not peripheral T cells. The Ly series of antigens has come into recent use because these antigenic determinants turn out to be a complex series of structures which immunologists can use to subdivide populations of T cells. The plasma cell (PC) antigen found on plasma cells and the mouse bone marrow lymphocyte antigen (MBLA) is present only on B cells. The murine histocompatibility antigen, the H-2 system, is similar to the HLA antigen system in man. These transplantation antigens are found both on B and T cells but do not give us an indication of the cells' functional capability.

One way to assess the functional ability of T and B cells is to activate them with agents which mimic the way antigens activate these cells. Phytomitogens are plant-derived proteins which selectively activate T or B cells. For example, when phytohemagglutinin (PHA) is added to spleen cells (a mixture of T and B cells), only T cells will be activated to become blast cells while B cells are unaffected. Blast transformation is one of the early steps involved in maturation of these cells after interaction with antigens. Another lectin which will specifically stimulate populations of T cells is Concanavalin A (Con A). Endotoxin, derived from Gram-negative bacteria, will specifically activate murine B cells.

Thymus and bone marrow derived cells are also uniquely susceptible to inactivation by commonly used therapeutic agents. B cells are more sensitive to steroids than T cells. T cells are more affected by antilymphocyte serum than B cells.

In the immune response to most antigens, T cells both regulate and help in the process of antibody production by B cells. Thymus derived cells alone can act as both effector and regulator cells in the development of cell mediated immune reactions; those reactions involved in the rejection of allografts and tumors. The bone marrow is the source of stem cells which seed the thymus and the Bursa equivalent for B cells in mammals. After a period of maturation in these primary lymphoid organs, T and B lymphocytes seed secondary lymphoid organs such as lymph nodes, spleen and gut associated lymphoid tissue. T and B cells have unique properties with respect to antigen binding receptors, cell surface antigens, response to mitogens and susceptibility to inactivation by various agents which make the study of their quantitative distribution and functional attributes possible. As more is learned about how these cells function, effective selective clinical manipulation of the immune response may become possible in man.

ANTIGEN RECOGNITION BY LYMPHOCYTES

Emil R. Unanue, M.D.

Department of Pathology
Harvard Medical School
Boston, Massachusetts 02115

The immune response represents a collaborative enterprise between various sets of lymphocytes and mononuclear phagocytes. The lymphocytes represent a heterogeneous population grouped into two major sets: The B class, representing the progenitors of antibody-forming cells, and the T or thymic-derived class, which includes various subsets exerting regulatory influences and mediating cellular immune reactions. It has been established, at least for the B cells, that antigen recognition takes place through molecules localized on their plasma membrane. The nature of the receptor molecules and their properties have been reasonably well documented. Controversy exists regarding the receptor for antigen on T lymphocytes. Insofar as the mononuclear phagocytes, it is thought that interaction with antigens takes place by means of various surface "receptors". Phagocytes have receptors for the Fc piece of IgG and for the third component of complement, enabling them to interact with antigen-antibody complexes; also, phagocytes may bind antigen by way of chemically uncharacterized sites on their surface.

We will consider in this paper antigen recognition by B lymphocytes where the information is more extensive. Recognition by T cells and macrophages will be analyzed briefly.

Antigen Recognition by B Cells

About ten years ago, immunologists had some thoughts on how immune recognition should take place but had little hard information on it. The biological nature of antigen recognition on B lymphocytes seems well established now, and the biological characterization of the process is well underway. Paul Ehrlich, in 1900, was the first to theorize about some of the events taking place in immune cells. He postulated that cells interacted with toxins via "side chains" that stemmed from protoplasm. As systemic immunity developed, "the cells became, so to say, educated or trained to reproduce the necessary side chains in ever increasing quantity" (1). "Antitoxins represent nothing more than side chains reproduced in excess during regeneration and, therefore, pushed off from the protoplasm, and so coming to exist in a free state." The scheme of Ehrlich was basically correct. We now know that B lymphocytes, the progenitors of antibody-forming cells, have Ig on their membranes as the recognition unit. As induction takes place and differentiation occurs, the B cell changes to an active secretory stage, the plasma cell. Fifty to sixty years later, however, sufficient advances in cellular immunology had taken place; and the questions began to be asked concerning the molecular nature of antigen recognition. In the late 1950's several investigators postulated the selective theories of antibody formation (2-4). It was thought that antibody formation resulted in a random fashion: An extension that such cells had on their surface a "cell-associated antibody" served to bind antigen and initiate the process. When antigen entered, it selected the cell having the specific receptors. As Burnett explained, "it is assumed that, when an antigen enters the blood as tissue fluids, it will attach to the surface of any lymphocytes carrying reactive sites which correspond to one of its antigenic determinants."

The other groups of theories for antibody formation were the instructional theories. These postulated that antibody was formed by having the antigen molecule as a template-the antibody molecule folded about the antigen, acquiring a complementary configuration (5). These theories have now been abandoned,as our understanding of the mechanisms of protein synthesis indicated that it was a process encoded in the genome of the cells. The specificity of an antibody results from the primary amino acid sequence of the variable region of the light and heavy chains of an Ig molecule. Antibody molecules can be unfolded by denaturing agents and lose their antibody combining capacity. Upon removal of the denaturing agents, the antibody molecule refolds in the absence of antigen and reacquires its antibody-binding site (6).

Furthermore, antibody is secreted in cells that do not contain antigen. In general terms, all the evidence now available points in the direction of the selective theories.

The selective theories were postulated at a time when the pioneering studies of Gowans and associates strongly indicated that lymphocytes were the cells responsible for the initiation of the response (7). However, at this time, no evidence of Ig associated with the lymphocyte surface could be found. Immunofluorescence of tissue smears or thin sections introduced by Coons and associates disclosed Ig in the cytoplasm of plasma cells but not on lymphocytes (8). The first indication of Ig associated with lymphocytes came from the results of experiments by Gell and Sell, who found that rabbit lymphocytes in culture transformed into lymphoblasts upon exposure to appropriate anti-Ig antibodies (9,10). They postulated that the immune reaction at the cell surface initiated the signal that led to the proliferation of the cell. They further indicated that the putative Ig did not derive from the serum. The direct visual demonstration of Ig came a few years later. It was shown to be on cell surfaces by immunocytochemical methods provided unfixed, live cells were reacted with appropriately labeled antibodies in suspension and then processed (11-14).

It is now accepted that Ig is the receptor for antigen on B cells, a fact clearly proven by experimental methods. Whether or not it is present on the thymic (T) cell population remains a matter of considerable debate and controversy. Using routine cytochemical methods of detection, Ig is found only on B cells and hence it can be used as a marker for this cell type.

The cytochemical methods to detect surface Ig using anti-Ig antibodies vary, depending on the nature of the visual marker attached to them. At the level of the light microscope, the one most commonly used method is immunofluorescence, using fluorescein isothiocyanate. Immunofluorescence has been found to be particularly useful in the routine identifications of surface Ig on B cells. Suspensions of viable cells are incubated with the appropriate fluorescent label, washed to remove the unbound fluorescent label, and examined immediately after fixation. Using immunofluorescence, surface Ig can be readily identified as discrete, irregular, speckled points of fluorescence. The patterns of immunofluorescence must be seriously taken into consideration. Surface Ig, when complexed with antibody, is readily mobile within the plane of the membrane, redistributing and forming aggregates of various sizes. These aggregates then coalesce into one pole, giving the appearance of a cap. This redistribution occurs extremely fast at 37°C and even at ambient temperature. Following patching and capping, cells rapidly interiorize the Ig-antibody complexes in vesicles. This stage can be distinguished by the change in fluorescent pattern to discrete round beads (14, 15).

A second method to detect surface Ig is autoradiography, employing I^{125}-labeled antibodies (16), which is more time consuming but much more sensitive than immunofluoresence. Autoradiography at light microscope levels was not found to be very suitable for analyzing the different patterns of reactivity.

A third method that has been employed consists of using suitably coated red cells as indicator cells. This method has been used extensively by Coombs and associates in studies on rabbit lymphocytes (16). Rabbit lymphocytes are incubated with an anti-Ig antibody in the presence of indicator red cells coated with subagglutinating amounts of rabbit anti-red cell antibody. The anti-rabbit Ig links the rabbit Ig-coated red cells to the Ig-containing B lymphocytes. The techniques using red cells as indicator cells are limited in their applicability and have been largely superseded by more direct and cytologically more precise methods.

Ig on lymphocyte surfaces have also been identified at the ultrastructural level by various kinds of methods. Three kinds of molecules have been attached to anti-Ig antibodies: large molecules such as ferritin, hemocyanin (17), or viruses (18), which can be easily visualized; enzymes such as horseradish peroxidase localized by the enzyme reaction product (18); and lastly, the use of radioactive materials such as I^{125}, identified by radioautography. The use of antibodies labeled with ferritin or viruses gives a more direct idea of the relationships between the labeled antibody and the surface Ig. However, some of the labeled molecules are very large and necessarily produce a large degree of steric hindrance, making precise mapping studies largely unsatisfactory.

Identification by Biochemical Methods

The biochemical methods used most extensively to study surface Ig are based on the procedure developed by Phillips and Morrison (19) to study red cell proteins (20-22). It consists of radiolabeling the surface proteins with I^{125} using lactoperoxidase as a catalyzer. The I^{125} is incorporated into those surface proteins having accessible tyrosines. The cell is then lysed, and the radiolabeled components are precipitated with a specific anti-Ig antibody; the precipitate is washed, dissolved, and then examined in SDS polyacrylamide gel electrophoresis. An alternative procedure that has been followed is to study the radiolabeled products following their spontaneous release from the cell (23). An alternative method to the direct radioiodination of surface proteins is to biosynthetically label Ig by culturing the cell in radioactive precursors- amino acids or sugars- and proceed to analyze the surface products (24).

Ig as a Marker of B Lymphocytes

Only a certain percentage of lymphocytes have Ig detectable on their surface. The early observations were made at the same time that the concept was being developed of two distinct functional classes of lymphocytes. In 1966, Claman, et al., made the observation in mice that mixtures of thymocytes and bone marrow cells transplanted into X-irradiated recipients synergized to make antibody, while each population by itself made a poor response (25). The idea of two cells interacting for antibody production was later pursued by Miller and Mitchell (26, 27), who showed that in such cell combinations the bone marrow population provided the precursor of antibody formation, while the thymocytes provided only a "helper" function. Immunoincompetent thymectomized animals contained the precursors of antibody formation but did not respond immunologically because of the absence of the helper cell population. Previous to these observations, studies in the chicken had indicated the presence of two primary lymphoid organs- the bursa of Fabricius and the thymus- controlling the development of antibody production and cellular immunity, respectively. How these two systems regulated the cell (or cells) of the response was not ascertained and had to wait for a few years (28,29). Experiments of Miller (30) using the mouse had shown the effects of thymectomy in impairing the development of cell-mediated immunities; no well-defined bursal equivalent has been defined in mammals (31).

It became immediately obvious that cells carrying surface Ig were the antibody-producing progenitors. Raff (32) first showed that the per cent of lymphocytes bearing surface Ig was increased in thymectomized animals or following treatment with anti-lymphocyte serum. Such treated animals were depleted of T cells and had a relative increase in Ig-positive cells. This observation was confirmed and extended in experiments showing that bone marrow cells but not thymocytes, when transplanted into X-irradiated recipients, gave rise to Ig-bearing cells (33). In the mouse an inverse relationship was easily demonstrated between cells belonging to the recirculating pool (i.e., the cellular compartment comprised of, or under the influence of the thymus, or cells bearing the θ alloantigen) and the number of Ig-bearing cells. For example, about three-fourths or more of blood lymphocytes, one-third in lymph nodes, and one-half in spleen, respectively, were Ig negative. Thymus lymphocytes did not have detectable surface Ig. Congenital athymic mice had a normal number of Ig-positive cells but no θ positive cells.

Studies in the chicken were particularly significant because of the presence of the bursa were found to contain surface Ig in contrast to those in the thymus which did not (34, 35). Bursectomy in the chicken, a procedure that ablates antibody production, led to a reduction of the Ig-positive cells of the spleens. In contrast, thymectomy produced a reduction of the Ig-negative spleen cells.

Studies in man in immune deficiency diseases have confirmed the observations first made in experimental animals. Most patients with X-linked aggammaglobulinemia have a marked decrease in primary and secondary lymphoid follicles and in plasma cells. These defects are accompanied by few, if any, Ig-bearing lymphocytes. In contrast, patients with congenital absence of the thymus or thymus lymphoplasia have absence of Ig-negative lymphocyte populations and a relative increase of the Ig-bearing cells.

These basic observations have been greatly extended in a series of functional studies leaving little doubt that the precursor of antibody-forming cells, the B cells, express Ig on their surface, while the thymocytes do not, within the limits of detectability of the immunocytochemical method. B cells are identified as those lymphocytes having detectable surface Ig, while the thymocyte and its derived cells lack detectable expression of Ig. The question of whether T lymphocytes carry some Ig molecules and the nature of the antigen receptor in these cells has been one that has given rise to considerable dispute which is beyond the scope of this review to analyze. There is general agreement that Ig molecules are not detected in T cells even with the most sophisticated cytochemical methods of detection. Our own experience was reviewed in 1973 (34). Biochemical methods have not resolved the controversy. Most investigators in repeated trials have not found any significant Ig from T cell membranes radiolabeled with lactoperoxidase. Marchalonis, et al. (36), however, claim finding large amounts. The results of Marchalonis and associates have been explained as resulting from small numbers of contaminating B cells or perhaps some Ig bound by cytophilia to some T cells. Speculation has arisen whether the Ig on T cells, if indeed present, are in very low numbers and/or partially hidden in the membrane; or that the receptor for antigen is a novel structure.

Ig Class

Although there are still some arguments concerning the main class of Ig represented on the B cell surface and on whether there is a single or multiple class at a given time, all the evidence tends to point to the following conclusions: 1) that IgM and IgD are the main classes of Ig represented on the cell surface; 2) that the number of cells expressing IgG- as a product of synthesis and not acquired from the serum- is low, although variations in number are found among species; and 3) that a B cell at a given time is restricted on the Ig class expressed- IgM and IgD are found usually together, but such is not the case with IgG; within the cells expressing IgG, only one allotype is found; finally, all Ig molecules of a given B cell have the same antibody-combining sites. The discrepancies found in the literature with regards to these points can be attributed to a large extent to the problem of cytophilic Ig. Although the bulk of Ig on the cell surface is a product of synthesis of the cell, some serum Ig may be found on the membranes, attracted by Fc-type receptors. Fc receptors are poorly defined surface structures which bind to the

Fc fragment of IgG. They are found most typically in monocytes and macrophages. B cells are known to have some Fc receptors.

IgM is without much doubt the major class of Ig of human peripheral blood B cells. Although some investigators have reported high percentage of IgG-bearing cells (reviewed by Warner, 37), recent studies point out that, in the majority of cases, this Ig is acquired from serum, although a certain number of IgG-bearing cells do exist.

Of great interest has been the recent observation that a great many lymphocytes bear IgD on their surfaces. Van Boxel et al. (38) first called attention to a higher percentage of IgD-positive cells in adult peripheral blood. Rowe, et al. (39), extended this observation by noting that most of the Ig in B cells in cord blood was, in fact, IgD. IgD is an Ig first discovered by Fahey and Rowe in a patient with multiple myeloma and found in normal serum in very low concentration (less than 0.04 mg per ml). About three-fourths of the peripheral blood lymphocytes have both IgM and IgD on their surfaces with only a few having one or the other Ig classes. The IgD is not acquired from the cell exterior and is made by the cell in culture (39). IgM and IgD are independent on the cell surface. Studies of chronic lymphocytic leukemia- in most cases a leukemia of B cells- indicate that in many instances lymphocytes will have both IgM and IgD with occasional cases having only one class. Other studies in man have indicated that in cells of patients with chronic lymphocytic leukemia all the light chains are of a single precursor.

The mouse and the rabbit have also been extensively studied. In mouse spleen the evidence by immunocytochemical analysis points to IgM as the main Ig on their membranes, although available amounts of cells having other classes have been found. Whether some of these cells have IgG on the basis of cytophilia- acquired from serum- is not clear. Several studies by Uhr, Vitetta and associates, Marchalonis, and Melchers and Andersson have indicated that IgM is the main Ig detectable by chemical means on the cell surface with small amounts of IgG or IgA chains. The IgM on the cell surface is mostly in the form of monomeric IgM. The IgM, however, that is secreted as the B cell differentiates into an active, secreting cell appears to be the classical 19S, pentameric type. The B cell with its monomeric IgM appears to release some of it to the outside environment, perhaps contributing this way to the pool of naturally occurring antibodies in the serum.

The question is being asked whether or not the mouse B cell also contains an IgD molecule similar to man. The lack of available anti-IgD antibodies makes it impossible to answer this using cytochemical techniques. Studies using lactoperoxidase labeling of the cell surface indicate the presence of another Ig on mouse B cells which is thought to be the equivalent of human IgD. Examination of SDS gels at a higher acrylamide concentration-7.5 to 10%-revealed the presence of a second Ig lighter in molecular weight than IgM (40,41). This Ig represents up to 40% of labeled Ig from splenic cells. This component is absent in B cells from neonatal mice. The IgD-like molecule appears at ten to fifteen days of age and increases until three months when it becomes the predominant cell surface Ig. Whether this Ig is truly the IgD of man is probably a correct speculation.

Lymphocytes appear to show, as do plasma cells, allelic exclusion; this is to say, they are committed to display Ig molecules of only one allotype and specificity. This was shown to be the case for the plasma cells which secreted molecules on only one class, allotype, and specificity (42,43). The point has been made, however, that some lymphocytes can exhibit both IgM and IgD at the same time and also that there can be a change in the class of Ig synthesized when it differentiates to a secreting cell, producing IgG. In other words, that there can be a switch of constant heavy chain genes apparently without a change in the genes coding for variable portions of the molecule. Precedence for this has been found in some cases of multiple myeloma, which may exhibit two sets of plasma cells, each secreting a different class of Ig but with the same variable regions.

The question of allelic exclusion has been examined in depth in the rabbit. Rabbit B cells lend themselves to this manipulation inasmuch as there are allotype markers controlled by different alleles for the light chain and for the heavy chain. Each allotype contains several allelic variants. Rabbit heterozygotes for Ig allotype cells are formed bearing one or the other but not both, i.e., each cell will express only one of its two allelic forms.

Redistribution and Capping

The fluid mosaic model envisions the plasma membrane as a two-dimensional solution of proteins within a fluid lipid bilayer (44). Depending on their chemical structure, the proteins in the membrane are embedded to variable degrees within the lipid layer, interacting in various ways with the lipid elements. Singer and Nicholson distinguished two groups of proteins-integral and peripheral - on the basis of their chemical interaction with the membrane. Peripheral proteins are weakly bound to the surface, easily dissociating by mild treatments. Integral proteins are those strongly bound, mostly by hydrophobic interactions with the membrane lipid, requiring detergents or organic solvents for isolation. The ionic and carbohydrate groups on integral proteins and lipids are located on the cell surface in contrast to the non-polar amino acid residues, which, by hydrophobic interaction, are in contact with the fatty acid chains of the lipid. The degrees to which an integral protein is embedded in the plasma depends on thermodynamic considerations. The model conceives that integral proteins have the freedom to translate themselves within the plane of the fluid lipid bilayer.

The manner in which Ig molecules are embedded in the plasma membrane has not been well defined. It is clear that the combining site of the molecule is readily available and capable of binding to antigen and so is a great part of the Fc fragment of the molecule. Indeed, antibodies to class determinants do react with surface Ig. There is some evidence suggesting that C-terminal end of the heavy chain may be partially hidden. The manner in which Ig interacts with membrane components is not clear, since no large hydrophobic segments are present in the molecule. Speculation has also arisen concerning the possibility that some other integral protein may serve as the attachment site. The possibility of an Fc receptor-like molecule acting as an anchoring unit has also been speculated.

Ig molecules, in agreement with the fluid mosaic model of membrane structure, are not rigidly anchored to the plasma membrane but are free to translate themselves within the plane of the membrane. The dramatic demonstration of the capacity of Ig to freely diffuse on the cell surface comes from studies using anti-Ig antibodies at 37°C (45-47). Lymphocytes incubated with anti-Ig antibodies, usually fluourescent labeled, at low temperatures, showed Ig molecules distributed throughout the surface in a thin, speckled pattern of fluorescence. As soon as the cell was warmed, however, the anti-Ig-Ig molecules formed large, irregular patches which rapidly coalesced into a single pole of the cell, forming caps of complexes. The whole phenomenon takes place extremely rapidly. Patching and capping have been studied in numerous cell types, including neutrophils, basophils, fibroblasts, etc. It appears to be a general phenomenon applicable to all cells. The first demonstration of diffusion of surface molecules came from the studies of Frye and Edidin (58) with heterokaryons. Surface antigens of two different cells were labeled with two different fluorochromes; after cell fusion, the patches intermixed, thus indicating that they were freely diffusing within the plane of the membrane.

The exact cytological events following binding of anti-Ig to lymphocytes are as follows: immediately after binding, small, irregular agglutinates are formed throughout the cell surface. They rapidly flow into a single pole, forming the cap. As the cell is capping, marked changes in cell shape take place. One of the earliest notable features is the development of a contraction involving the area right under the cap. Microfilaments have been found associated with the area of the cap molecules. At this time, the cell proceeds to exhibit translatory motion of a limited distance. These changes in cell shape and translatory motion can be rapidly generated and appear to be influenced by the levels of cyclic nucleotides in the cell. The complexes in the cap area are then interiorized by pinocytosis. The cap area has been found to be approximately opposite the Golgi area of the cell. The pinocyte vesicles flow into the centrosphere area and some fuse with lysosomes. It is surprising that the small B cell, with its paucity of lysosomal enzymes is perfectly capable of degrading the interiorzied complexes. Some of the complexes (10% to 20%) are shed off into the extracellular milieu during the phase of pinocytosis. Following these events, the lymphocyte is found bare of surface Ig. Upon culture, new molecules are reexpressed on their membrane within a few hours. If the ligand-receptor event is stimulatory, the cell differentiates into antibody-secreting cells.

The factors involved in patching and capping of Ig and other macro-molecules in lymphocytes have been studied quite extensively. The process is complex, involving, not only surface events but also the participation of cytoplasmic factors. First, patching and capping require a cross-linking ligand. That is to say, to initiate the micro-patching and agglutination as well as the flow into the cap, one requires that the surface Ig molecules be linked by a multivalent ligand. A monovalent anti-Ig, for example, will not produce any dramatic changes in the distribution of Ig. A cross-linking ligand has been thought to be also necessary for rapid endocytosis. Temperature is also a critical factor. Capping takes place at temperatures over 18 to 20°C, with an optimum at 37°C. Temperature may be critical with respect to the density of the lipid plasma membrane, which, at lower temperatures, would restrict the flow of macro-molecules. Low temperatures will also influence capping by lowering metabolism.

The sequence of events can be divided into energy-dependent and energy-independent events. The first event, patching, is not dependent on metabolic energy; but the second, capping, is highly dependent on it. Capping involves an active process by part of the cell and does not represent a simple, passive agglutination of complexes. The nature of the energy-dependent step involved is not clear but could be associated with the activation of microfilaments and microtubules, which may generate the force that drives the patches to one pole. The involvement of these organelles has been studied mostly by using pharmacologically active drugs.

What is the distribution of Ig on the cell surface prior to reaction with any ligand? The attempts to map surface Ig have used anti-Ig antibodies labeled with electron-dense markers. Distribution and mapping studies must be carried out by making two-dimensional maps of the cell surface, either by examining freeze-etched or whole-surface replicas. Recently, Abbas, et al. (49), published a study using entirely monovalent antibodies and the freeze-etched method. Murine B cells were labeled first with a fluorescein conjugate of a monovalent antibody to fluorescein conjugated ferritin. The pattern of Ig of cells fixed at 0°C or prefixed with paraformaldehyde was that of small microclusters forming an irregular, interconnecting network. The pattern of distribution was analyzed statistically, comparing it with an expected random distribution. It was apparent that the distribution of Ig sites was non-random, implicating a certain degree of organization of this protein on the plasma membrane. Attempts to elucidate the nature of micropatching have not clarified the issue. It is possible that the microclustering may result from secondary chemical interactions on the plasma membrane.

Binding of Antigen to Surface Ig

A function of Ig on the cell surface is to bind antigen molecules, a process essential to the stimulation of the lymphocyte. Studies of antigen binding by B cells have been made by morphological and functional techniques. Both approaches indicate that indeed the B cell interacts with antigen molecules via its Ig receptors; furthermore, they indicate that this binding is restricted to a few lymphocytes found in an individual prior to the entrance of antigen, in accordance with clonal selection theories. Direct antigen binding assays, therefore, support the conclusion that the response is restricted to the clones of lymphocytes having specificites for that antigen.

The use of highly radioactive antigen was first introduced by Sulitzeanu and associates (50). Lymphocyte suspensions were incubated with highly radioactive bovine serum albumin, washed extensively, and processed for autoradiography. It was found that a small percentage of small lymphocytes were binding the radioactive antigen. This observation was rapidly confirmed by other investigators, the following conclusions being made: 1) the cells binding antigen are small and medium-sized lymphocytes; 2) antigen binding can be decreased markedly by treatment of the cells with anti-Ig antibodies, indicating that the binding occurs via surface Ig; 3) lymphocytes binding antigen are found prior to antigen stimulation and increase in number during the immune response; 4) the lymphocytes that bind to antigen are essential to the expression of immunity, and their removal abrogates the response; and 5) antigen is redistributed on the cell surface in the same way described for surface Ig.

Several kinds of experiments point to the functional significance of antigen-binding cells. Lymphoid cells can be passed to columns having antigen attached to an insoluble matrix. Those lymphocytes bearing the specific receptors bind to the antigen and are retained in the column, therefore, depriving the efferent cell population of reactive cells (51). A second approach is the so-called "suicide" experiment first reported by Ada and Byrt (52) and Humphrey and Keller (53). Lymphocytes incubated with highly radioactive antigens are washed and then tested for their capacity to develop an immune response. The interaction with highly radioactive antigen apparently kills the cloned specific cells which are then unable to mount a response but do so to unrelated antigen.

B Cell Maturation and Stimulation

The distribution and metabolism of surface Ig varies among B cells, reflecting, in part, the state of maturation of the cell. All the evidence points out that the B lymphocyte evolves from a stage having little or no surface Ig to a second stage morphologically that of a small, medium-sized lymphocyte having variable amounts of Ig on its membrane with little active secretion and few rough endoplasmic reticulum to a fully developed secretory stage having relatively smaller amounts of surface Ig but secreting large amounts of it. This latter stage corresponds morphologically to the large lymphocyte-plasmablast, plasma cell stage in which the cell contains large amounts of rough endoplasmic reticulum. The B cell starts by synthesizing Ig entirely to function as a receptor for binding antigen, a process which is necessary to drive the cell to secretory stage; as the cell is stimulated and differentiates, it no longer requires Ig to serve as antigen receptor but instead exports Ig to the outside environment. Morphological studies on the sequence from a small, inactive B cell to the differentiated, fully secretory cell have been made on lymph nodes of animals undergoing immune response; but in these, the whole sequence of the reaction is difficult to ascertain. Some of the most informative morphological analyses supporting the sequence of differentiation have been made using cells following stimulation by mitogens.

There is a difference among lymphocytes with regard to the biochemical behavior of Ig. Small B lymphocytes, presumably in an active, nonstimulated stage, contain the bulk of synthesized Ig (about 90%) on their surface membranes, releasing small amounts of it into the outside medium in the form of 8S IgM. It has been speculated that the monomeric IgM released by inactive B lymphocytes contributes to the pool of natural antibodies found in serum. In contrast, endotoxin-stimulated cells have an increased synthesis of IgM, a great part of which is secreted in its polymeric 19S form. Large lymphocytes found in spleens of mice also secrete IgG. The whole sequence of change has been studied in detail following endotoxin stimulation.

The presence or absence of surface Ig can also be used to study the maturation of B lymphocytes. These studies have been mainly in mouse bone-marrow cells and in the bursa of the chicken. Mouse bone marrow is known to contain many rapidly dividing lymphocytes without any surface Ig. Kinetic studies suggest that these rapidly dividing cells are stem cells that may rapidly differentiate to cells containing surface Ig which then exits to peripheral lymphoid tissue (54). During their development in the bone marrow, the early B cells do not contain the C3 receptors found in B cells of spleen and lymph nodes, although they do have Fc receptors. Studies of the ontogenetic development of murine B cells indicate a stage in which B cells also lack C3 receptor (55, 56). Of great interest are recent observations indicating that these very early B cells are rapidly made tolerant upon exposure to antigen or anti-Ig reagents. Nossal and Pike (57) exposed in vitro bone marrow culture to small amounts of antigen and found that these cells, in contrast to spleen cells, were unable to respond to a subsequent strong immunological stimulus. In our laboratory, Sidman has found that brief exposures of the early B lymphocytes to anti-Ig rapidly inactivates them so they are no longer able to resynthesize Ig (58). Similar results have been obtained by Raff, et al. (59), using an in vitro culture system. Hence, the overall evidence suggests different stages in the maturation from a stem cell having no surface Ig to an early differentiated stage with surface Ig- no C3 receptor and an easy target for inactivation by ligands- to a more fully mature cell ready to be selected by antigen for stimulation and further differentiation. Studies in the chicken are discussed below.

The relationship between Ig displayed on the surface and that synthesized by the cell upon antigenic challenge has been the subject of debate. The results so far available have been conflictive and have not settled this question which remains open. One thought is that the early B cell bearing IgM (and IgD) is driven to IgG synthesis upon antigen stimulation. A second hypothesis championed by

Cooper and Lawton and their associates postulated that the IgM-bearing cells go through a sequence of antigen-independent maturational stages into IgG and then IgA-bearing cells (60). In the adult individual, Ig G secretion is viewed as resulting from direct stimulation of the IgG-bearing cell.

Several lines of evidence are in favor of the IgG-secreting cell deriving from an IgM-bearing precursor. Suggestive evidence comes from the observations that the bulk of the Ig-bearing B cells have IgM (and IgD) on their membrane yet upon antigen stimulation are driven to IgG secretion. However, inasmuch as some IgG-bearing cells do exist, these could explain, in part, the results. The most direct evidence comes from two series of experiments. In one, antibodies to μ chain were found to inhibit development of IgM, IgG, and IgA antibody-producing cells in cultures of murine spleen cells exposed to sheep red blood cells (61). In cultures of primed spleen cells, i.e., cells from mice previously immunized and having immunologic memory, anti -μ treatment affected much less the development of IgG and IgA cells. These results can be interpreted to mean that, upon antigen stimulation, the B cells shift the production of their heavy chain constant genes without altering the specificity of the variable region genes. Antigen stimulation then results in plasma cells secreting various classes of Ig as well as generation of memory cells now bearing not only the μ chain but γ and α chain.

Conclusion

In this review, we have considered several aspects of the receptor for antigen in B class of lymphocytes. Several points appear to be well grounded on a firm experimental basis. Clearly, the lymphocytes that represent the progenitors of plasma cells have Ig on their surface, and this antibody serves as an antigen receptor. The lymphocyte line goes through several stages of differentiation from a small cell bearing Ig but not secreting to a fully secreting cell- the plasma cell. Differentiation takes place as a result of antigen stimulation usually involving complex interactions involving the cooperative cells like the T cells and the macrophages. These cellular interactions have not been analyzed here. We have some good ideas on the disposition, mobility, and fate of surface Ig when complexed with ligand. The phenomenon of capping is a dramatic demonstration of surface mobility and has served as a basis to study surface cytoplasmic interactions. However, the control of ligand receptor complexes and the exact nature of the biochemical signals that derive from these interactions have yet to be determined. Insofar as the class of Ig on the membrane, there is general agreement that IgM and IgD in man are the main classes; but the exact number of IgG-bearing cells is controversial. It has become clear recently that B cells carry Fc receptors and that some serum Ig can bind to it. Caution needs to be exercised, therefore, in the execution and determination of immunocytochemical analyses. The evidence is compelling that the Ig on the cell surface is restricted, having specificity for one antigen and showing allelic exclusion. Also, the evidence is quite good for a switch in class of Ig as the cell differentiates to a secreting stage. Clearly, one area of future investigation concerns the biochemical and cellular events following interaction of surface Ig with antigen in the presence or absence of cooperative events.

REFERENCES

1. Ehrlich, P. (1900). Proc. Royal Soc. (London) 66: 2456.
2. Burnet, F.M. (1959). "The Clonal Selection Theory of Acquired Immunity." Vanderbilt University Press, Nashville.
3. Jerne, N.K. (1955). Proc. Nat. Acad. Sci. (USA) 41: 849.
4. Talmage, D. W. (1957). Ann. N.Y. Acad. Sci. 70: 82.
5. Pauling, L. (1940). J. Amer. Chem. Soc. 62: 2643.
6. Haber, H. (1964). Proc. Nat. Acad. Sci. (USA) 52: 1099.
7. Gowans, J.L. (1970). Harvey Lect. 64: 87.
8. Coons, A.H., Leduc, H.E., and Connolly, J.M. (1955). J. Exp. Med. 102: 49.

9. Sell, S., and Gell, P.G.H. (1965a). J. Exp. Med. 122: 423.

10. Sell, S., and Gell, P. G.H. (1965b). J. Exp. Med. 122: 923.

11. Raff, M.C., Steinberg, M., and Taylor, R.B. (1970). Nature 225: 553.

12. Pernis, B., Forni, L., and Amante, L. (1970). J. Exp. Med. 132: 1001.

13. Rabellino, E., Colon, S., Grey, H.M., and Unanue, E.R. (1971). J. Exp. Med. 133: 156.

14. Coombs, R.R.A., Gurner, B.W., Janeway, C.A., Wilson, A.B., Gell, P.G.H., and Kelus, A.S. (1970). Immunol. 18: 417.

15. Taylor, R.B., Duffers, W.P.H., Raff, M.C., and de Petris, S. (1971). Nature New Biol. 233: 255.

16. Unanue, E.R., Perkins, W.D., and Karnovsky, M.J. (1972). J. Exp. Med. 136: 885.

17. Karnovsky, M.J., Unanue, E.R., and Levanthal, M. (1972). J. Exp. Med. 136: 907.

18. Aoki, T.H., Wood, H.A., Old, L.J., Boyse, E.A., de Harven, E., Landis, MP.P., and Stackpole, C.W. (1971). Virology 65: 858.

19. Phillips, D.R., and Morrison, M. (1970). Biochem. Biophys. Res. Commun. 40: 284.

20. Bauer, S., Vitetta, E.S., Sherr, C.J., Shenkin, I., and Uhr, J.W. (1971). J. Immunol. 106: 1133.

21. Marchalonis, J.J., Cone, R.E., and Santer, V. (1971). Biochem. J. 124: 921).

22. Vitetta, E.S., Bauer, S., and Uhr, J.W. (1971). J. Exp. Med. 134: 242.

23. Marchalonis, J.J., and Cone, R.E. (1973). Transplant. Rev. 14: 3.

24. Melchers, F., and Andersson, J. (1973). Transplant. Rev. 14: 76.

25. Claman, H.N., Chaperon, E.A., and Triplett, R.F. (1966). Proc. Soc. Exp. Biol. Med. 122: 1167.

26. Miller, J.F.A.P., and Mitchell, G.F. (1968). J. Exp. Med. 128: 801.

27. Mitchell, G.F., Grumet, C.F., and McDevitt, H.O. (1972) J. Exp. Med. 135: 126.

28. Glick, B., Chang, T.S., and Jaap, R.G. (1956). Poultry Sci. 35: 224.

29. Warner, N.L., and Szenberg, A. (1962). Nature 196: 784.

30. Miller, J.F.A.P. (1961). Lancet 2: 748.

31. Good, R.A. (1972). Harvey Lect. 67: 1.

32. Raff, M.C. (1970). Immunol. 19: 637.

33. Unanue, E.R., Grey, H.M., Rabellino, E., Campbell, P., Schmidtke, J. (1971). J. Exp. Med. 133: 1188.

34. Rabellino, E., and Grey, H.M. (1971). J. Immunol. 106: 1418.

35. Hudson, L., and Roitt, I.M. (1973). Eur. J. Immunol. 3: 63.

36. Marchalonis, J.J., Cone, R.E., and Atwell, J.L. (1972). J. Exp. Med. 135: 956.

37. Warner, N.L. (1974). Adv. Immunol. 19:1.

38. van Boxel, J.A., Stobo, J.D., Paul, W.E., and Green, I. (1972). Science 175: 194.

39. Rowe, D.S., Hug, K., Forni, L., and Pernis, B. (1973). J. Exp. Med. 138: 965.

40. Melcher, U., Vitetta, E.S., McWilliams, M., Lam, M.E., Phillips-Quagliata, J.M., and Uhr, J.W. (1974). J. Exp. Med. 140: 1427.

41. Abney, E.R., and Parkhouse, R.M.E. Nature (London) New Biol. 252: 600.

42. Pernis, B., Chiappino, G., Kelos, A.S., and Gell, P.G.H. (1965). J. Exp. Med. 122: 853.

43. Cebra, J.J., Colberg, J.E., and Dray, S. (1966). J. Exp. Med. 123: 547.

44. Singer, S.J., and Nicholson, G.L. (1972). Science 175: 720.

45. Unanue, E.R., and Karnovsky, M.J. (1973). Transplant. Proc. 14: 184.

46. Unanue, E.R., Engers, H.D., and Karnovsky, M.J. (1973). Fed. Proc. 32: 44.

47. Loor, F., Forni, L., and Pernis, B. (1972). Eur. J. Immunol. 2: 203.

48. Frye, C.D., and Edidin, M. (1970). J. Cell Sci. 7: 313.

49. Abbas, A.K., Ault, K.A., Karnovsky, M.J., and Unanue, E.R. (1975). J. Immunol. 114: 1197.

50. Sulitzeanu, D. (1971). Current Topics in Microb. Immunol. 54:1.

51. Wigzell, H., and Anderson, B. (1969). J. Exp. Med. 129:23.

52. Ada, G.L., and Byrt, P. (1969). Nature 222:1291.

53. Humphrey, J.H., and Keller, H.U. (1970). "Developmental Aspects of Antibody Formation and Structure. (J. Sterzl and I. Riha, eds.) Vol. II, p. 485, Academic Press, New York.

54. Osmond, D.G., and Nossal, G.J.V. (1974). Cell. Immunol. 13:117.

55. Gelfand, M.C., Elfenbein, G.J., Frank, M.M., and Paul, W.E. (1974). J. Exp. Med. 139:1125.

56. Sidman, C.L., and Unanue, E.R. (1975). J. Immunol. 114:1730.

57. Nossal, G.J.V., and Pike, B.L. (1975). J. Exp. Med. 141:904.

58. Sidman, C.L., and Unanue, E.R. (1975). Nature 257:149.

59. Raff, M.C., Owen, J.J.T., Cooper, M.D., Lawton, A.R. Megson, M., and Gatherings, W.E. J. Exp. Med. 142:1052.

60. Cooper, M.D., Keightley, R.G., Wu, L.Y.F., and Lawton, A.R. (1973). Transplant. Rev. 16:51.

61. Pierce, C.W., Solliday, S.M., and Asofsky, R.J. (1972). J. Exp. Med. 135:675.

GENETIC CONTROL OF IMMUNE RESPONSIVENESS: A DYNAMIC INTERPLAY BETWEEN GENES, CELLS AND MOLECULES

David H. Katz, M.D.

Harvard Medical School, Dept. of Pathology

Boston, Massachusetts 02115

INTRODUCTION

The immune system is one of the most intricate of all bodily systems, paralleling in many respects the endocrine system in terms of the multiplicity of functions required of it for maintaining homeostasis and integrity of each individual's health. Both systems exert control over discrete functions at great distances within the body by virtue of circulating components capable of performing their role(s) at sites quite removed from their point of origin, and in this sense they display a level of versatility not found in most other multicellular organ systems. They differ, however, in one important respect: the endocrine system encompasses several distinct endocrine organs each endowed with specific, and limited, functional capabilities; each organ is comprised of distinctive cell types and architecture, and the complexity of the system itself stems from the intricate communications network existing among these organs (and their respective target tissues) mediated in large part by the hormonal products generally unique to each of them. In contrast, the immune system consists of relatively few distinct organs-- i.e. thymus, spleen, bone marrow and lymph nodes-- which are composed of relatively few distinct cell types. Although it is true that there are numerous lymph nodes throughout the body, each one is generally structured in much the same manner as all the rest and appear to owe their multiplicity to the strategic nature of their different locations more so than any differences in general function.

Accordingly, the complexity of the immune system has evolved from an intriguing communications network established between the components of the system, designed in such a manner as to permit a multiplicity of effects to arise from relatively few distinct cell types. This has been accomplished by development of sophisticated regulatory mechanisms allowing either enormous amplification or contraction of a given response depending on the needs of the individual. Under normal circumstances, the system functions remarkably well to maintain effective defenses against foreign agents and against aberrant native cells which may have undergone neoplastic transformation as a consequence of either normal random mutational events or secondary or exogenous oncogenic influence. Many other circumstances exist, however, in which abnormalities in one or more components of the system result in some form of breakdown in the network manifested clinically in various ways and levels of severity.

In this presentation, I will attempt to give an overview of the immune system, with particular emphasis on the regulatory mechanisms involved in the responses developed by the system and the genetic control of such regulatory mechanisms. At the outset, I should forewarn the reader that much of what I will say reflects my own personal perspectives about the system, and hence should not be necessarily construed as incontrovertible. Indeed, one of the remarkable features of the immune system is that its cellular and molecular components are so enormously complex that evolution has built into the system an incredible degree of flexibility--rarely, does it seem, has the system created a single pathway to an end with no alternative avenue to take when a biological detour becomes advantageous. Therefore, it appears most appropriate to assume that only a few absolutes exist in the immune system. Moreover, time has taught those of us actively working in the field that the system is considerably smarter than man himself as evidenced by the still numerous unanswered questions concerning it.

COMPONENTS OF THE IMMUNE SYSTEM

As stated above, the intricacies of the immune system stem from the remarkable communications network established between the components of the system. These components, as depicted in Fig. 1 are essentially genes, cells and molecules; the interplay between them is reciprocal and circumscribed, thus laying the foundations of the regulatory mechanisms controlling the system. A similar reciprocal and circumscribed relationship exists between the major cellular components of the system (Fig. 2).

A. Cells

The major cellular components of the immune system are the macrophages and lymphocytes (Fig. 2). Macrophages are themselves very versatile in the functions they perform in a variety of immune responses (see ref. 1 for review). Although not themselves specific for any given antigen, they perform a crucial role in concentrating and presenting antigens to lymphocytes; in particular, they appear to determine, in some way, whether and which T lymphocytes will be induced to stimulation and function by various antigens. Moreover, macrophages secrete several biologically active mediators capable of regulating the type and magnitude of lymphocyte responses by either enhancing or suppressing cell division and/or differentiation. All of this is in addition to their functional capabilities as the major phagocytic cells of the reticulo-endothelial system, clearing the system of debris including molecular aggregates, foreign bacteria and dead cells.

The lymphocytes represent the specific cellular component of the system, specificity being conferred upon such cells by virtue of the existence of antigen-specific receptors on the surface membrane of each immunocompetent cell. The nature of receptor specificity is highly specialized in that each different clone of lymphocytes expresses its own unique specificity; the origin of such specialization--i.e. whether genetically inherited or induced by somatic mutation--is not defined as yet, and remains a subject of debate. Moreover, the nature of antigen receptors on the two major classes of lymphocytes may differ. Thus, it is well established that surface immunoglobulin (Ig) molecules serve as the antigen receptors for bone marrow-derived

FIGURE 1

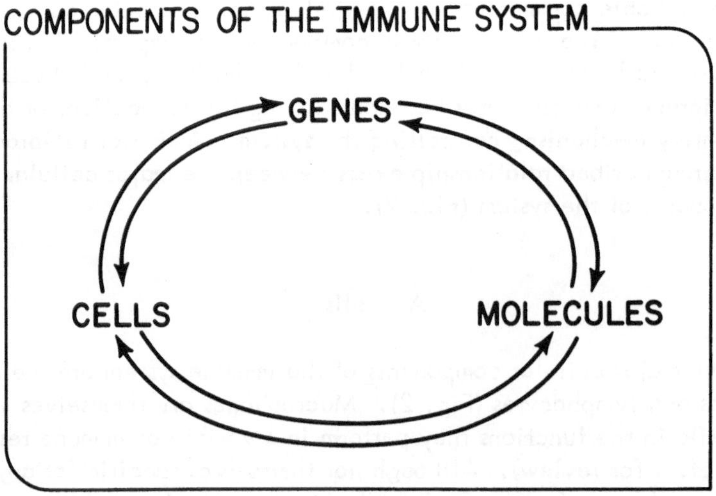
COMPONENTS OF THE IMMUNE SYSTEM
GENES
CELLS
MOLECULES

FIGURE 2

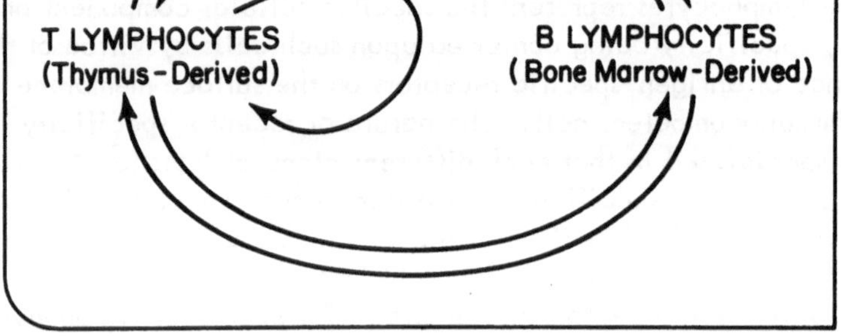
CELLS OF THE IMMUNE SYSTEM
MACROPHAGES
T LYMPHOCYTES
(Thymus-Derived)
B LYMPHOCYTES
(Bone Marrow-Derived)

or B lymphocytes (indeed, this is one of the few absolutes in Immunology); the molecular nature of antigen receptors of thymus-derived or T lymphocytes is still controversial and mounting evidence indicates that it is probably not Ig, at least certainly not of the conventional type functioning as receptors on B cells. More detail on this subject has been presented elsewhere in this Symposium by E.R. Unanue.

The two classes of T and B lymphocytes have very distinct functional capabilities, which are summarized in Table I. T lymphocytes do not themselves produce circulating antibodies, nor do they give rise to antibody-secreting cells. They can be subdivided into two major functional categories, based upon studies in the mouse in which the most extensive investigations have been made (reviewed in refs. 2,3).

1) Regulatory T lymphocytes are those cells functioning to either facilitate or amplify ("helper" cells) or suppress ("suppressor" cells) the responses of other T lymphocytes or of B lymphocytes. These functions appear to be mediated by distinct subpopulations of T cells since helper and suppressor T cells have been found to differ in size and most importantly, in certain cell surface antigenic markers.

2) Effector T lymphocytes are those cells responsible for cell-mediated immune reactions such as delayed hypersensitivity (DH) responses, rejection of foreign tissue grafts and tumors, and elimination of virus-infected cells. The latter two responses involve the participation of cytotoxic T lymphocytes, (CTL) commonly referred to as "killer" cells; also involved in responses to foreign tissues are T cells which undergo rapid proliferation in mixed lymphocyte reactions (MLR). The MLR cell and CTL can be distinguished from one another by the presence of different surface markers; likewise, CTL can be distinguished from DH cells on the basis of surface markers.

However, DH, MLR and helper T cells possess similar surface markers and it remains to be established by other criteria whether or not these are functions performed by the same or distinct T cell subpopulations (although some evidence exists to suggest helper and DH cells are different). The same is true for CTL and suppressor T cells, which are indistinguishable in their surface antigen phenotype.

Categorization of functional subpopulations of B lymphocytes is most readily done on the basis of different Ig classes synthesized (Table I). B lymphocytes give rise to cells synthesizing and secreting all classes of circulating Ig--i.e. IgM, IgG, IgA and IgE -- and the respective B cell precursors for these antibody-forming cells are $B\mu$, $B\gamma$, and $B\alpha$. The situation is a bit more complex in the sense that the earliest progenitors of antigen-specific B cells possess receptors of the IgM class; more mature B cells possess both IgM and IgD whereas the most mature precursor B cells (or perhaps "memory" B cells) express IgD alone on their surface (4). It appears, therefore, that the B cell precursors of IgM, IgG and IgA - secreting cells may derive from the same subline of B lymphocytes; precursors of IgE - secreting cells appear to represent a distinct subline. Memory B cells are functionally important for the development of rapid secondary, or anamnestic, antibody responses upon subsequent antigenic exposure; these cells can be distinguished from unprimed B lymphocytes by several features including tissue distribution, size, migratory properties, and certain surface antigen differences. There is not hard evidence for the existence of regulatory B lymphocyte analogous in function to regulatory T lymphocytes, although the discovery of such cells in the future would not be entirely surprising. The capacity of antibody molecules themselves to specifically regulate responses by the process of "antibody feedback" is well documented.

B. Molecules

The second major component category is comprised of the molecules of the immune system (Table II). Historically, the Ig system has been the longest recognized molecular component and until recent years regarded as the only one of functional importance; it is now clear that other molecular species are equally important in their functional roles either as effectors or regulators of various immune responses. The Ig system is the paradigm of specificity (insofar as antigens are concerned) among the molecules of the system and subserve different biological functions depending on the heavy chain class. With the exception of IgD, which appears to serve mainly as a cell-bound antigen receptor, all of the classes of Ig listed circulate in the serum and hence can potentially operate at great distances from their point of origin, this itself being an enormously efficient process particularly

Table I

FUNCTIONAL SUBPOPULATIONS OF LYMPHOCYTES

I. T LYMPHOCYTES

A. REGULATORY T LYMPHOCYTES

1. Helper Cells
2. Supressor Cells

B. EFFECTOR T LYMPHOCYTES

1. Delayed Hypersensitivity (DH)
2. Mixed Lymphocyte Reactivity
3. Cytotoxic T Lymphocyte (CTL or "Killer" Cells)

II. B LYMPHOCYTES

A. PRECURSORS OF ANTIBODY - FORMING CELLS
B , B , B , B ,

B. MEMORY CELLS

C. ? REGULATORY B LYMPHOCYTES

TABLE II

MOLECULES OF THE IMMUNE SYSTEM

IMMUNOGLOBULINS (Antibodies) - Products of B Lymphocytes

IgM IgG IgA IgE IgD	1) Receptors of B Cells 2) Secretory Products of Plasma Cells

BIOLOGICALLY ACTIVE MEDIATORS - Products of T Lymphocytes and Macrophages

MIF, etc.

HISTOCOMPATIBILITY ANTIGENS

COMPLEMENT

PHARMACOLOGIC MEDIATORS - Histamine, Serotonin, etc.

when one considers that each single cell can produce hundreds of thousands of Ig molecules.

The other category of molecules capable of functioning in a highly regulatory manner are the various biologically active mediators produced by T lymphocytes and macrophages. Some of these, such as migration inhibition factor (MIF) which is active in delayed hypersensitivity reactions, have no inherent specificity for antigen, although induction of the T cell responsible for synthesizing MIF occurs via antigen-specific receptors. Hence, this is the example par excellence of specificity in induction but non-specificity in effector function, of which several types of examples exist in T lymphocyte responses. On the other hand, recent studies have revealed the existence of of antigen-specific biologically active non-Ig mediators produced by T lymphocytes and capable of exerting either suppressive or enhancing regulatory influences on other lymphocytes. Interestingly, these T cell factors as well as certain non-antigen-specific T cell factors have been found to possess histocompatibility antigen determinants demonstrating an integral role of the histocompatibility system in regulatory mechanisms controlling immune responses as originally suggested by other studies (reviewed in refs 3 and 5). The histocompatibility antigens also serve as major transplantation antigens, although it is clear that this was not involved in the evolutionary selective pressures maintaining the system's integrity.

The complement system in itself a highly intricate network of component molecules each exerting distinct biological or chemical functions (reviewed in 6), and the activities of numerous pharmacologic mediators such as histamine, serotonin and similar substances in various immunological phenomena cannot be overstated in their importance (reviewed in 7).

C. Genes

In general terms, there are three "families" of genes that are integral to the function(s) of the immune system (Table III). Of course, central to the major function of B lymphocytes are the genes responsible for directing synthesis of Ig molecules. The situation here is genetically unique in that the Ig gene system is the only one

TABLE III

GENES OF THE IMMUNE SYSTEM

A. IMMUNOGLOBULIN GENES

1. Variable (V) Region Genes (Antibody Combining Site)
2. Constant (C) Region Genes (Biological Function)
3. Light (L) Chain - Kappa, Lambda
4. Heavy (H) Chain - M, G, A, E, D

B. HISTOCOMPATIBILITY GENES

1. Major and Minor Transplantation Antigens (Graft and Tumor Rejection)
2. Complement Components
3. Interations with Viruses

C. I-REGION GENES

1. Control of T Cell Recognition (? T Cell Receptor)
2. Disease Susceptibility - Resistance to Viruses; Allergic Disorder
3. Involved in B Cell Differentiation
4. Control of T Cell - Macrophage Interactions
5. Control of T Cell - B Cell Interactions
6. Biologically Active Mediators (T Lymphocytes and Macrophages)
7. Major Antigens Responsible for Mixed Lymphocyte Reactivity and Graft-versus-Host Reactions (Ia Antigens)

known to involve the participation of two discrete structural genes in the production of a single polypeptide chain. Thus, a structural gene for the variable (V) region -- i.e. the specific combining site of the molecule -- integrates with another structural gene for the constant (C) region of the molecule (determines biological function of the molecule, such as the capacity of IgE to bind to most cells) to form a single polypeptide chain comprised of V and C regions. Each intact Ig molecule consists of four chains, two identical light (L) chains and two identical heavy (H) chains (the latter determine Ig class -- i.e. IgM, IgG, IgE, etc. -- of the molecule), so that there are V_L and V_H genes as well as C_L and C_H genes. Putting these together in proper fashion to make a functional Ig molecule is in itself an extremely complex affair (reviewed in ref. 8).

Another gene family that plays a crucial role in the immune system is that concerned with the histocompatibility system. In man and in the mouse, where this system has been most thoroughly studied, the major histocompatibility gene complexes are known as HLA and H-2, respectively. Both HLA and H-2 have been shown to consist of several distinct regions, the genes of which are responsible for distinct functions. As illustrated in Figure 3, the H-2 complex, which is located in a small segment of chromosome 17 of the mouse, consists of seven regions and sub-regions. The H-2K and H-2D regions on either end contain the genes responsible for the major transplantation antigens present on essentially all cells of the body and readily detected serologically with appropriate antibodies. The K and D genes are also the major antigens against which cytotoxic T lymphocytes are directed in graft rejection responses following tissue transplantation. Furthermore, it has recently been shown that the products of K and D genes interact with cytopathogenic viruses, in a manner yet to be determined, to create new antigenic determinants capable of inducing cytotoxic T cell responses effective in eliminating such virus-infected cells from the individual; evidence also exists indicating that chemical modifications of the K and D antigens results in a similar process. These findings suggest the operation of an efficient surveillance mechanism generated by alterations of originally normal "self-antigen" components on cell surfaces which in turn induce immune reactions to eliminate such "altered" cells. The S region contains structural genes responsible for synthesis of certain components of the complement systems, and the G region contains genes controlling synthesis of certain alloantigens present on erythrocytes.

The I region genes thus far have been shown to be the most versatile in terms of their functional relationships to immune responses. In the mouse there are three well defined sub regions, I-A, I-B, and I-C (Fig. 3)., and recent studies indicate the possible existence of at least two others (I-F and I-J). Contained within one or more of these sub-regions are genes controlling an individual's capacity to respond (or not) to various antigens including different viruses and hence susceptibility to certain diseases (immune response or Ir genes), cell interactions (CI) genes regulatinginteractions between macrophages, T cells and B cells, genes involved in synthesis of certain biologically active mediators produced by T cells, and structural genes for I-region-associated (Ia) antigens which are the major antigens stimulating mixed lymphocyte reactions and graft-versus-host activity (reviewed in ref. 9). Ia antigens are also involved in cell interactions and B lymphocyte differentiation in ways that are still unresolved. It is not established at present whether distinct genes are responsible for the various functions just mentioned or whether such functions are controlled by relatively few genes; the latter possibility would not be very surprising since many of these functions are closely related to one another, as will be discussed in the following section. Similar functional distinctions have been assigned to different regions of the HLA gene complex of man (reviewed in ref. 10).

REGULATORY INTERACTIONS IN IMMUNE RESPONSES

One of the major breakthroughs in our understanding of the immune system has been the discovery of its intricate network of regulatory interactions. Stemming largely from the work in the mid-1960's of Claman and Miller and Mitchell and their co-workers in this country and Australia, respectively, which pointed out the requirement for T-B cell interactions for development of antibody responses (reviewed in refs. 2 and 3), our persepctive in this regard has been greatly enlarged so that now, in the mid-1970's, we can view such regulatory interactions as reflecting a dynamic interplay between all of the various genes, cells and molecules of the immune system (Table IV).

Hence, the genes of the system control synthesis of 1) antigen

TABLE IV

REGULATORY INTERACTIONS IN IMMUNE RESPONSES

I. GENES

A. Control Receptor Recognition of Antigen by Cells
B. Initiate Synthesis of Biologically Active Molecules
C. Determine and Regulate Effectiveness of Cell-Cell Interactions

II. CELLS

A. Macrophage - T Cell Interactions; Macrophage - B Cell Interactions
B. T Cell-T Cell Interactions ⟶ Cell-Mediated Immunity
C. T Cell-B Cell Interactions ⟶ Antibody Production

III. MOLECULES

A. Serve as Specific Antigen Receptors on Lymphocyte Surface Membranes
B. Regulate Cell-Cell Interactions
C. Circulating Antibodies - Effector Function and Feedback Regulation
D. Enhance or Suppress T Cell and/or B Cell Functions

FIGURE 3

REGIONS AND SUBREGIONS OF THE *H-2* GENE COMPLEX

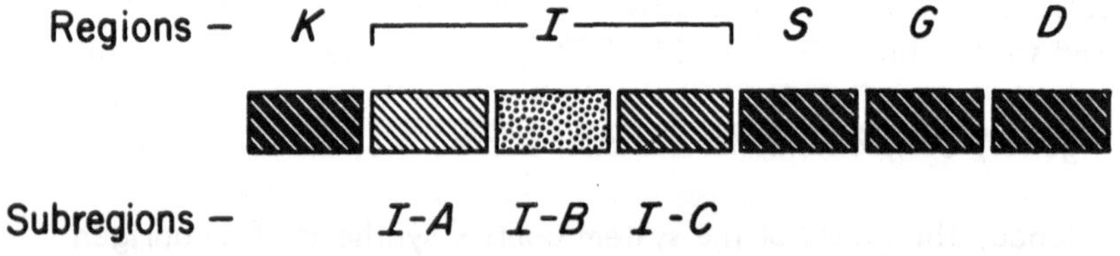

receptors on T and B cells, 2) the Ig products of B cells and the biologically active T cell mediators responsible for regulating quality and magnitude of immune responses, and 3) the capacity of macrophages, T cells and B cells to interact and the effectiveness of such interactions. The cells of the system are interdependent upon one another so that the development of either cell-mediated or humoral immunity is regulated by a program of essential interactions between T cells, macrophages and B cells (see also Fig. 2). The consequences of such cell interactions depend, in turn, on the molecules serving as either specific antigen receptors on surface membranes of lymphocytes or as secretory products of such cells (or macrophages) which exert effector functions (i.e. antibody molecules) or participate in regulating cell interactions and/or cell differentiation.

The net effects of such regulatory interactions between the genes, cells and molecules of the immune system span an entire spectrum ranging from enhancement at one end to suppression at the other. The qualitative and quantitative response occurring at any given time reflects the net effect of this extremely dynamic interplay among the these components.

GENETIC CONTROL OF IMMUNE RESPONSIVENESS

When we speak of genetic control of immune responses, we are referring to a concept defined on the basis of original work in this area which demonstrated the association of certain genes with the capacity of certain individuals to develop responses to well-defined antigens (reviewed in refs. 11 and 12). The different categories of genes pertinent in this regard are summarized in Table V. The crucial association was found to be between such genes, known as immune response or Ir genes, and the major histocompatibility gene complex (MHC) more specifically, the I region of the MHC. Ir genes have been found in essentially all species, including man, and appear to be involved in the recognition of antigens and the events concerned with specific T cell induction and function. They are inherited in simple Mendelian fashion as autosomal dominant traits; in certain cases, it has been recently discovered that two genes are responsible for permitting responses to develop to a given antigen. Hence, absence of either one of the genes, or both, results in inability of the individual to respond to the antigen in question (11, 12).

More recently, it has been discovered that genes present in the I-region of the MHC also govern the development of specific suppressor T cells. In contrast to the situation with Ir genes, in which absence of a gene or genes results in non-responder status of the individual to the antigen in question, the absence of a specific Is gene (or genes) allows a response to occur to the antigen essentially dissociated from any regulatory influence of suppressor T cell activity. Although studies in this area have only recently begun, it is conceivable that genetic defects in the Is gene system may have greater clinical relevance than those of the Ir system, particularly in areas of autoimmunity and allergic disorders.

Another area of genetic control of immune responsiveness concerns the regulation of most effective cell-cell interactions. It has been demonstrated that the interactions between macrophages and T cells and between T cells and B cells involves cell surface molecules, termed cell interaction (CI) molecules, whose synthesis is controlled by CI genes located in the I region of the MHC (reviewed in refs. 3,5, and 11). In addition, biologically active T cell mediators in the mouse capable of either enhancing or suppressing immune function, have been shown to possess antigenic determinants of gene products of the I region of H-2 (i.e. Ia antigens); it is not known as yet whether the genes responsible for synthesis of such molecules and the CI genes are identical or distinct or, moreover, whether these are the same or different from Ir and Is genes.

The most recent genetic association has been that related to cytopathogenic viruses and the major serologically-defined transplantation antigens--i.e. the H-2K and H-2D region gene products. For convenience, I have termed the relevant genes antigen-interaction (AI) genes to denote the fact that, in some as yet undefined manner, the products of these genes interact with viruses or chemicals on the cell surface to undergo some form of physical alteration which in turn is recognized as foreign by host lymphoid cells. The necessity for this alteration of "self" antigens in order to induce immunity against the invasive agent is presently obscure, but obviously of immense practical importance to maintenance of host integrity. It is quite likely that the alteration of "self" in this way plays a

TABLE V

GENETIC CONTROL OF IMMUNE RESPONSIVENESS

I. IMMUNE RESPONSE (Ir) GENES

A. Control antigen recognition and stimulation in T lymphocytes -- i.e. absence of a gene prevents response.

B. Presence or absence may determine susceptibility to certain etiologic agents such as viruses, or predisposition to development of certain diseases of unknown etiology such as multiple sclerosis, ankylosing spondylitis, myasthenia gravis--perhaps even insulin-dependent diabetes.

II. IMMUNE SUPPRESSION (Is) GENES

A. Control stimulation of specific suppressor T lymphocytes--i.e. absence of a gene allows response.

B. Presence or absence may determine susceptibility to certain etiologic agents such as viruses, or predisposition to development of certain diseases of unknown etiology such as multiple sclerosis, ankylosing spondylitis, myasthenia gravis--perhaps even insulin-dependent diabetes.

III. CELL INTERACTION (CI) GENES

A. Control most effective macrophage- T lymphocyte interactions.

B. Control most effective T-B and T-T cell interactions.

C. Produce molecules active in enhancing and suppressing immune responses.

IV. ANTIGEN-INTERACTION (AI) GENES

A. Control interactions between certain antigenic determinants (particularly viruses and transplantation antigens on the cell surface).

B. Determine "immunological surveillance" against new antigenic determinants such as tumor-specific transplantation antigens.

C. ? Protect against "self-recognition".

protective role against spontaneous or induced neoplastic transformation, and may also be pertinent to maintaining homeostasis against inadvertent self-recognition and autoimmunity.

EXAMPLES OF CLINICAL CIRCUMSTANCES REFLECTING ABERRANT GENETIC AND REGULATORY CONTROL OF IMMUNE RESPONSES

There is at present a lengthy list of diseases in which primary or associated immunologic abnormalities exist. Perhaps the most thoroughly investigated of these are the primary immunodeficiency diseases associated with genetic defects in immunoglobulin synthesis and/or cell-mediated immune functions (reviewed in refs. 13 and 14). In Table VI, I have listed only a few representative examples of other possible clinical manifestations of aberrant genetic and regulatory control of immune responses, some of which have been documented, the rest of which are more speculative. I have deliberately focused this list on defects associated with regulatory T cell functions, since it is this area about which only little is presently known, but which may turn out to be extremely far reaching in clinical medicine in the coming years.

Defects in suppressor T cell activity can be manifested as either an excess over normal or relatively deficient. In either case, the net effect is one of upsetting the normal homeostasis usually dependent on the appropriate balance of suppressor and helper T cell activity. Already documented is the existence of excessive (or aberrant) suppressor T cell activity in certain forms of acquired hypogammaglobulinemia in man (15). Thus, peripheral blood lymphocytes from such patients fail to synthesize and secrete immunoglobulins in tissue culture under appropriate conditions of stimulation capable of inducing Ig synthesis in cultures of normal human lymphocytes. The defect, however, is not intrinsic to the B cells in these cases since it has been shown that removal of T lymphocytes from the cultured population enables the isolated B cells to synthesize and secrete Ig. Moreover, addition of patients' T cells to cultures of normal human lymphocytes inhibits the latter cells from synthesizing and secreting Ig. Hence, the presence and activity of an aberrant population of suppressor T cells is phenotypically expressed as hypogammaglobulinemia in such

TABLE VI

EXAMPLES OF CLINICAL CIRCUMSTANCES REFLECTING ABERRANT

GENETIC AND REGULATORY CONTROL OF IMMUNE RESPONSES

I. DEFECTS IN SUPPRESSOR T CELL FUNCTION

A. Excess Suppressor Activity
1. Certain forms of acquired hypogammaglobulinemia.
2. ? Immunodeficiency of ageing.
3. ? Immunodeficiency associated with certain neoplastic disorders - i.e. Hodgkin's disease.

B. Deficient Suppressor Activity
1. IgE-mediated allergic disorders - i.e. ragweed allergy.
2. ? Certain autoimmune states.
3. ? Malignancies of lymphoid cell clones - i.e. plasmacytomas, leukemia.

II. DEFECTS IN HELPER T CELL FUNCTION

A. Excess or Inappropriate Helper Activity
1. ? Certain autoimmune states.

B. Deficient Helper Activity
1. Congenital thymic deficiencies - i.e. DiGeorge syndrome.
2. Susceptibility to certain diseases of viral etiology.

patients.

More speculative is the possibility that the immunodeficiency of ageing may reflect, at least in part, a similar condition of excess suppressor T cell function; this, however, could be a relative excess based in part on varying degrees of deficiency in helper T cell activity. Similarly, one could envisage the immunodeficiencies associated with certain neoplastic diseases to result from a relative excess of suppressor T cell function. A prime candidate for this possibility is the deficiency in T cell-mediated immunity frequently observed in patients with Hodgkin's Disease. Indeed, recent studies have indicated that exposure of peripheral blood lymphocytes from anergic patients with active disease to the anti-helminthic drug Levamisole in vitro enables such cells to respond to certain phytomitogens known to induce DNA synthesis in T cells (16). This suggests that anergy in such patients may reflect the existence of an inhibitory mechanism preventing T cell responses in vivo rather than any absolute T cell deficiency. Suppressor T cells would be a strong candidate for effecting such a mechanism.

Deficient suppressor T cell activity is perhaps best exemplified in the IgE-mediated allergic disorders of man. Studies in our own laboratory and in that of Dr. Tada in Japan and Dr. Ishizaka at Johns Hopkins have indicated that the development of high titers of IgE antibodies following antigen exposure occurs in conditions where suppressor T cell activity is quite low; the converse is true in the presence of normal suppressor cell function. Moreover, we have obtained recent evidence suggesting that genetic mechanisms underlie this relative deficiency in suppressor cell function in animals prone to develop high IgE antibody responses. The absence or relative deficiency of suppressor cell activity may be involved in the pathogenesis of certain autoimmune disorders and/or in malignancies of lymphoid cell clones such as certain leukemias and multiple myeloma. These disorders could well reflect escape of various components of the immune system from normal regulatory controls.

Similar speculation can be entertained about the existence of inappropriate helper T cell activity in the pathogenesis of some autoimmune diseases. In this case, one could envisage non-specific or cross-reactive helper cell activity generated by exogenous agents or adjuvants which in turn results in the loss of normal self-tolerance. The deficiencies of helper (as well as effector) T cell functions associated with congenital abnormalities such as DiGeorge Syndrome are well documented. On the more speculative side, although experimental support exists, is the association of susceptibility to certain viral diseases to genetic defects in the capacity to mount effective immune response to such agents. The relationship of such defects to development of malignant diseases of possible viral etiology remains to be established.

INDUCTION OF CELLULAR INTERACTIONS IN IMMUNE RESPONSES

Despite intensive efforts by many investigators around the world, a precise delineation of the manner in which lymphocytes are activated and the mechanisms of cell-cell interactions has yet to be made. Nevertheless, considerable information has been obtained which permits a circumstantial view of the probable events involved. I have depicted certain of these possibilities in Figures 4 and 5.

A view of T-T cell interactions in the development of cell-mediated immune response is schematically illustrated in Fig. 4. The example employed is that of responses to a virus which is shown to be expressed on the cell surface of a macrophage (although other cells would be suitable as well) in association with a histocompatibility (H) molecule; the precursor of the cytotoxic T lymphocyte (CTL) has specific receptors directed presumably to the virus-H molecule complex. Notice the release of biologically active factors from the macrophage which in turn may act on regulatory helper and/or suppressor T cells (whether or not the latter cells manifest any specificity for the virus itself or virus-H molecule complex is unknown). The helper T cell, once activated, is capable of interacting with the CTL precursor presumably via cell-interaction (CI) molecules located on the cell membrane; this event may occur either by direct cell-cell contact or via soluble mediators, as illustrated, or both. Nonetheless, the consequences of such interactions are to facilitate the final differentiation of the CTL precursors to mature effector cells and/or to memory cells. The suppressor T cell may interfere with these events at one or more of three possible points indicated by the

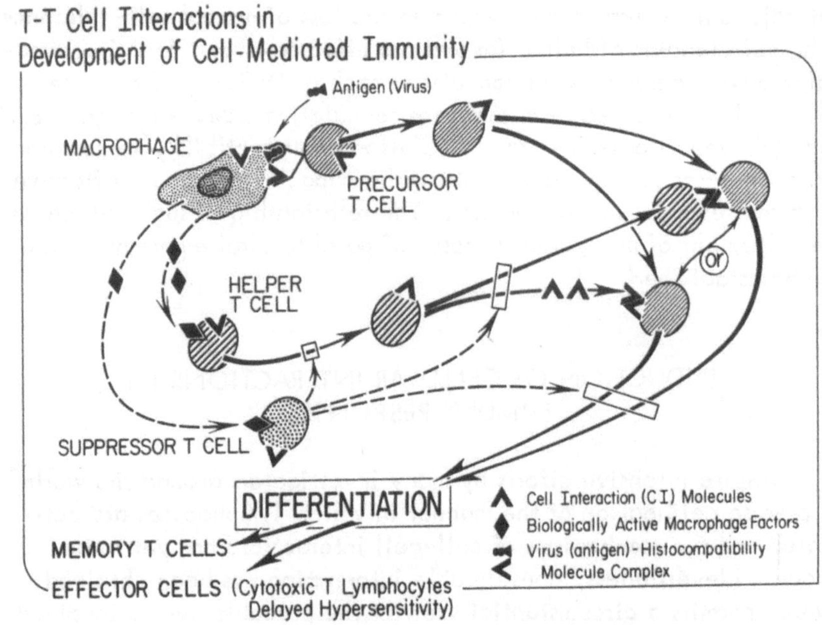
T-T Cell Interactions in
Development of Cell-Mediated Immunity
Antigen (Virus)
MACROPHAGE
PRECURSOR
T CELL
HELPER
T CELL
or
SUPPRESSOR T CELL
DIFFERENTIATION
Cell Interaction (CI) Molecules
Biologically Active Macrophage Factors
Virus (antigen)-Histocompatibility
Molecule Complex
MEMORY T CELLS
EFFECTOR CELLS (Cytotoxic T Lymphocytes
Delayed Hypersensitivity)

FIGURE 5

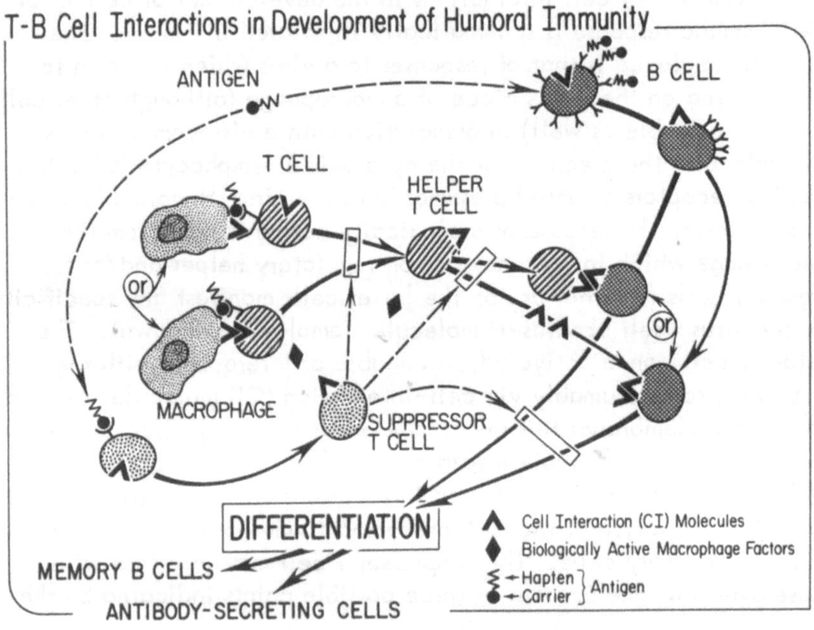
T-B Cell Interactions in Development of Humoral Immunity
ANTIGEN
B CELL
T CELL
HELPER
T CELL
or
or
MACROPHAGE
SUPPRESSOR
T CELL
DIFFERENTIATION
Cell Interaction (CI) Molecules
Biologically Active Macrophage Factors
Hapten
Carrier
Antigen
MEMORY B CELLS
ANTIBODY-SECRETING CELLS

broken arrows: first, in the activation of helper T cells; second, in the actual function of the helper T cell in terms of its facilitating interactions with the CTL precursor; or third, in the actual differentiation of the precursors to effector cells (either before or after interaction of the precursors with helper cells).

A similar scheme for T-B cell interactions in the development of antibody responses is illustrated in Fig. 5. The antigen here is a hapten-carrier conjugate in which case the carrier determinants are recognized by T cells and the haptenic determinants by the B cells. Macrophage presentation of antigen appears to be particularly favorable for inducing helper T cells; whether the helper T cell recognizes carrier determinants alone or a complex of carrier determinants associated with H molecules (analogous to the CTL precursor in Fig. 4) is a subject of current interest and discussion. In any event, there is clearly an important role of macrophage - associated CI molecules in the induction of specific helper T cell function. Once activated the helper T cell interacts with B cells specific for the hapten (which have previously interacted with hapten determinants via their surface Ig receptors), to facilitate the differentiation of such cells to mature effector cells--i.e. antibody secreting plasma cells, or to memory cells. These interactions may occur either by direct cell-cell contact of via soluble T cell factors, as illustrated. As in the case of T-T cell interactions, suppressor T cell activity may interfere with this sequence by preventing either helper T cell induction or function in interactions with B cells or by directly inhibiting B cell differentiation.

CONCLUSION

This brief overview has been directed to bringing a broad perspective to the dynamic interplay among the genes, cells and molecules of the immune system which serve to maintain a homeostasis between the individual and its environment. One of the main advantages of the complexity of the system is the flexibility inherent in it to allow compensatory or alternative routes to be taken when certain defects, transient or permanent, occur in one or more of its components. Nevertheless, certain defects alone or in combination may occur resulting in deleterious primary or secondary consequences. It is the aim of many of us working in this area to elucidate the nature of such defects and to ascertain therapeutic alternatives to restore such homeostasis in applicable circumstances. This is a foreseeable reality in the near future.

Acknowledgments

I am grateful to Charlene Small for excellent assistance in preparation of the manuscript. Work conducted in my laboratory is supported by NIH Grant AI-10630.

REFERENCES

1. Unanue, E.R. 1972. The regulatory role of macrophages in antigenic stimulation. Advanc. Immunol. 15: 95.

2. Katz, D.H., and B. Benacerraf. 1972. The regulatory influence of activated T cells on B cell responses to antigen. Adv. Immunol. 15:1.

3. Katz, D.H. 1976. Lymphocyte Differentiation, Recognition and Regulation. Academinc Press, Inc., New York.

4. Vitetta, E.S., and J.W. Uhr. 1975. Immunoglobulin-receptors revisted. Science 189: 964.

5. Katz, D.H., and B. Benacerraf. 1975. Hypothesis. The function and interrelationships of T cell receptors, Ir genes and other histocompatibility gene products. Transpl. Rev. 22: 175.

6. Colten, H.R. 1976. Biosynthesis of complement. Adv. Immunol. 22: 67.

7. Becker, E.L. and P.M. Henson. 1973. In vitro studies of immunologically induced secretion of mediators from cells and related phenomena. Adv. Immunol. 17: 94.

8. Natvig, J.B. and H.G. Kunkel. 1973. Human immunoglobulins: classes, subclasses, genetic variants, and idiotypes. Adv. Immunol. 16:1.

9. Shreffler, D.C., T. Meo and C.S. David. 1976. Genetic resolution of the products and functions of I and S region genes of the mouse H-2 complex. In The Role of Products of the Histocompatibility Gene Complex in Immune Responses. D.H. Katz and B.Benacerraf, editors. Academic Press, New York. Page 3.

10. Van Rood, J.J., A. Van Leuwen, A. Termijtelen and J.J. Keuing. 1976. The genetics of the major histocompatibility complex in man, HLA. In The Role of Products of the Histocompatibility Gene Complex in Immune Responses. D.H. Katz and B. Benacerraf, editors. Academic Press, New York. Page 31.

11. Benacerraf, B. and D.H. Katz. 1975. The histocompatibility-linked immune response genes. Adv. Cancer Research 21: 121.

12. Benacerraf, B. and D.H. Katz. 1975. The nature and function of histocompatibility-linked immune response genes. In Immunogenetics and Immunodeficiency. B. Benacerraf, editor. Medical and Technical Publishing Co., Ltd. London. p. 117.

13. Rosen, F.S. 1975. Immunodeficiency. In Immunogenetics and Immunodeficiency. B. Benacerraf, editor. Medical and Technical Publishing, Co., Ltd. London. p. 221.

14. Good, R.A. 1973. Immunodeficiency in developmental perspective. The Harvey Lectures, Series 67:1.

15. Waldmann, T.A., S. Broder, M. Durm, M. Blackman, and B. Meade. 1975. Supressor T cells in immunodeficiency. In Immune Depression and Cancer. G.W. Siskind, C.L. Christian and S.D. Litwin, editors. Grune and Stratton, New York. p. 20.

16. Ramot, B., M. Biniaminov, Ch. Shoham, and E. Rosenthal. 1976. Effect of Levamisole on E-rosette-forming cells in Hodgkin's Disease. New England J. Med. 294: 809.

ALPHA TO OMEGA ON THETA BEARING LYMPHOCYTES: IMMUNOREGULATION BY T CELLS

Richard K. Gershon and Charles M. Metzler, M.D.

Yale University School of Medicine, Dept. of Pathology

310 Cedar Street, New Haven, Conn. 06510

INTRODUCTION

Within a very short period after a foreign substance enters the body, two opposing forces are sent into action, one positive and the other negative. The positive force has as its main goal the production of substances which will attack the invader and neutralize and/or kill it. These attacking forces are extremely heterogenous but can be subdivided into two main categories, cell-mediated and humoral immune responses. Cell-mediated immunity consists of various types of blood cells which have the ability to either actively or passively recognize the specific nature of the foreign invader and to kill it. Humoral immunity consists predominantly of antibodies, which bind to foreign substances with exquisite specificity. Antibodies are divided into several classes (i.e. IgM, IgG with its many subclasses, IgE, IgA, etc.), depending on particular antigenic (and other) markers found in the constant region of their heavy chains. In addition to binding to foreign substances, antibodies of some of the classes can also bind to cells. Cell-bound antibodies thus provide some aspect of specificity to cell-mediated immune responses and therefore, serve as a "bridge" between the cellular and humoral arms of the immune response.

The negative force which is set into motion when the foreign substance enters the body is one whose job is to stop or suppress production of active immune responses. Under ideal conditions, an adequate cellular or humoral response is usually made before suppressive influences come into play, and the suppressor's job is then simply to regulate the level of the response. However, under some circumstances, the appropriate immunoregulatory feedback system breaks down and either too vigorous or too poor a response is made. In this short review article, we would like to discuss some of the forces and cell interactions which determine how the immune response knows which of its attacking factors to make and how it knows when sufficient numbers are made. We will also discuss some of the forces which cause the suppressive part of the equation to be overly predominant, thus resulting in a depressed or insufficient immune response. Perhaps an appropriate way to start this review is to divide the immune system into two parts: one which is thymus dependent, and one which is not.

THYMUS INDEPENDENT RESPONSES

The thymus independent portion of the immune response consists predominantly of IgM antibodies and low affinity IgG antibodies. This part of the immune response is quite primitive both phylogenetically and ontogenetically (for more detailed review of this aspect see 1). There is, however, some recent evidence suggesting that there might also be a phylogenetically and ontogenetically quite advanced component to the thymus independent response. This possibility is based on preliminary data from studies on a mutant mouse called the CBA/N mouse which seems to have a B cell maturation defect and fails to make some thymus independent antibodies, which all other strains of mice can make (2). These recent findings help explain some paradoxical observations made previously by Birger Andersson who studied the immune response to a "classic" thymus independent antigen polyvinylpyrollidone (PVP) (3). He noted that immature B cells made a poor thymus independent response to this antigen, but that this response could be improved by the addition of T cells. Mature B cells on the other hand, made a better thymus independent response to PVP, but their response was shut off by the same number of T cells that helped the response of the immature B cells. Assuming that there are two types of thymus independent B cells, and that there are regulatory T cells (see below) which sense the activity of the cells that they are regulating by feedback mechanisms, these observations of Andersson now seem less paradoxical.

In any case, thymus independent responses are usually mounted against non-protein antigens which have many repeating determinants, such as polysaccharides and PVP, which are generally poorly catabolized. These antigens are particularly predominant on Pneumococci and related bacteria. The thymus independent response is regulated in two ways: (1) Through IgM feedback and/or (2) through the activity of suppressor T cells (which will be discussed in more detail below).

Other portions of the immune response which presently seem to be thymus independent to a large degree, are the activity of non-thymus derived killer cells (K cells), and some elements of the reticulo-endothelial system. In the near future, however, it will probably be found that these primitive thymus independent responses are altered, modified and improved by T cell activity.

THYMUS DEPENDENT RESPONSES

It would seem that the most phylogenetically advanced portion of the immune response, from both the humoral and cell-mediated aspects, is T cell dependent. Responses under T cell control would include production of high affinity IgG antibodies, and specialized antibodies such as IgA and IgE. In addition, many forms of cell-mediated immunity are under T cell control, including classical delayed hypersensitivity reactions, the more recently described delayed type hypersensitivity (DTH) response called cutaneous basophil hypersensitivity, graft versus host responses, graft rejection, and other more esoteric subdivisions of these major responses. How do these T cell dependent responses work? They work through the combined interaction of three major classes of cells: T cells, B cells and macrophages. There seems to be considerable heterogeneity in all three of these cell populations. At present little is known about functional heterogeneity among B cell and macrophage populations; therefore, we will not discuss them any further in this article, except to emphasize that there undoubtedly is considerable heterogeneity within them, and it is quite important that future work elucidate the precise functions of all subsets within these two major classes of cells. However, recent work has defined the role of several T cell subsets, and we will focus the remainder of the article on this particular subject.

T CELL SUBSETS

Not until 1967 was it first recognized that T and B cells interacted in the production of antibody; prior to that time the two systems were thought to be independent. Following this, it was only a short time before it became recognized that there were also interactions between subsets of T cells. The two subsets of T cells which were first identified became known as T1 and T2 (4). Basically T1 was an immature cell, did not recirculate, and therefore was richly represented among T cells in the spleen and thymus. The T2 cell was more mature, did recirculate, and therefore was more richly represented among T cells in peripheral lymph nodes and in the thoracic duct lymph. The less mature T1 cell was more sensitive to drugs such as cortisone and cytoxan, and to irradiation and adult thymectomy. The more mature T2 cell was a longer-lived cell than T1. The precise nature of the interactions between these two types of T cells was difficult to define because they lacked stable markers.

Following the discovery of T and B cell interactions, as the positive or synergistic interactions between T1 and T2 cells were being worked out, it also became apparent that there was another functionally distinct subset of T cells whose main function was to suppress the immune response (1). This subset became known as suppressor T cells. Although the evidence was much less convincing, it also seemed that there were interactions between T1 and T2 cells in the generation of suppressor T cells, and that the actual suppressor cell was in the T2 class (1). Thus the T1, T2 sub-division clearly did not divide T cells by function into helpers and suppressors.

During this historical developmental period of immunology the literature can be quite confusing. This is probably due to the complex nature of the interactions between the T cell subsets and to the fact that there were no stable markers on any of the T cell subsets which researchers could use as handles to isolate the cells and determine their functions. Thus the breakthrough work of Cantor and Boyse in 1975 (5,6), defining T cell subsets by stable antigenic markers, has enabled the immunologic community to make much more sense out of what previously seemed to be confusing morass of conflicting data.

Basically, Cantor and Boyse have defined distinct T cell subsets using antisera directed against the products of genetic loci which are expressed as antigens on some but not all peripheral T cells of inbred mouse strains and are called differentiation antigens. Production of these antisera was possible since different inbred strains of mice bear different alleles at these loci, and mice of one strain can therefore be immunized with cells from another. These antigens are thus analogous to standard Ig allotypes (see below). These differentiation antigens are part of a series called Ly and so far three Ly loci have been identified. There are four Ly subsets. One subset contains all three of the Ly antigens as well as the TL antigen and is called Ly 1,2,3 TL^+, this cell is found only in the thymus. Another cell lacks the TL antigen, but contains all three of the Ly antigens and this cell is called Ly 1,2,3. It is found in small numbers in the thymus and represents 100% of the T cell pool of mice less than 2 weeks of age and about 50% of the T cell pool of young adult mice. The percentage of these cells in aged mice has not yet been determined; but it is probably significantly lower than 50%, since all available evidence suggest that this cell is the predominant cell of the T cell subset previously called T1, which wanes in number with age. The other two T cell subsets are both predominantly in the T2 class. One expresses only the Ly 1 antigen and is therefore called Ly 1; it represents approximately 30% of the T cell pool of young adult mice. So far this subset has been found to only have positive or helper effects, which includes helping other T cells to differentiate into killer cells. Killer T cells belong to the fourth T cell subset called Ly 2,3, which express both Ly 2 and Ly 3 antigens. Ly 2,3 cells represent somewhere between 5-10% of the T cell pool of adult mice. Besides being killer cells, cells of this latter subset are also suppressor cells, suppressing not only antibody formation but DTH responses as well. No stable markers have yet been found which can distinguish between the two functions of the Ly 2,3 subset (i.e. killer and suppressor). In fact, some workers think that these two functions may turn out to be inseparable, but a great deal more work is required before this conclusion can be definitely expressed.

MIGRATORY CHARACTERISTICS OF LYMPHOCYTE SUBSETS

An important question the above discussion may provide an answer to is why some subsets of cells have the ability to recirculate (that is to leave the blood, enter the lymph and then return to the blood), whereas other subsets seem inherently incapable of leaving the blood. The answer to this question may be obtained from some of our recent work on DTH. We have found that the predominant cells in the DTH lesion, macrophages which have recently arisen in the bone marrow of the challenged animal, require the activity of vasoactive amines to leave the blood and enter the DTH site. Another population of cells, almost certainly long-lived recirculating T cells of the Ly 1 subset, can leave the blood without the requirement for vasoactive amine activity. Thus it might be that the recirculating cell can freely pass the very tight junctions of specialized venule endothelium, perhaps by emperipolesis as suggested by Gowans and Marchesi (7). When it meets the triggering antigen in the tissues outside of the blood, it releases factors which fire mast cells and/or basophils which in turn release vasocative amines. The amines then open the specialized venule endothelial junctions to a sufficient extent to permit other cells, which normally do not recirculate, to align.

TIPPING THE BALANCE: HELP VERSUS SUPPRESSION

For physicians trying to manipulate the immune response for the benefit of patients, the question of prime importance is: What are the factors which can result in either improving or suppressing the immune response (depending upon need)? This question can be phrased more academically by asking: What are the factors which favor the development of helper or suppressor T cells? The important factors so far identified include the following:

(1) The use of adjuvants

These substances tend to favor the production of helper cells. The mechanism(s) through which they do so is not entirely clear at the moment. It is clear, however, that most adjuvants are non-specific T cell stimulators. In addition, there is sufficient data to speculate on another important mechanism through which they act; which is by generating resistance in the helper cell to the activity of the suppressor cell population. For example, it has clearly been shown that after an encounter with antigen, helper cells either mature or differentiate into a state where they become relatively resistant to the activity of the suppressor cell and that adjuvants favor this non-specific T cell differentiation (8). Thus, by including adjuvants along with an immunizing dose, one can generate considerably more helpers cells before the suppressor cells take over and stop the response.

(2) Physical form of the antigen

For unknown reasons, but almost certainly due to some role of the reticulo-endothelial system, presentation of the antigen in a particulate form favors generation of help over suppression. The mechanism through which it does so is probably closely related to the one through which adjuvants work. Thus presentation of antigen in a soluble form is more likely to result in a preponderance of suppression or a net increase insupression, while presentation of the antigen in a less soluble or aggregated form will favor the net balance of help. We use the term "net balance" to indicate that, although one may get considerably more suppressor cells when using adjuvants or particulate antigens, the productions of helpers, which have considerable resistance to the effects of suppressor cells, will outpace the production of suppressors. On the other hand, when using soluble antigen one may get poorer production of suppressor cells but even poorer production of helper cells, so that the net balance favors suppression, even though the total number of suppressor cells generated is less.

(3) Antigen dose

Both sub-optimal and supra-optimal doses of antigen favor the net increase of suppressor cells over helper cells, probably by different mechanisms. Sub-optimal doses seem to activate fewer suppressor cells, but not counter-balancing helper cells; whereas supra-optimal doses activate large amounts of both helpers and suppressors, but suppression predominates. In the latter situation preliminary evidence indicates that excess antigen directly blocks or interfers with helper or other productive activity to a lesser extent than it interferes with suppressor activity.

(4) Feedback signals

It has clearly been shown that increased activity of either B cells or helper T cells results in increased production of suppressor cells (9). It has been suggested (but not proven) that this mechanism results from inducing the Ly 1,2,3 cells to either differentiate into Ly 2,3 suppressor cells or (less likely) to increase the activity of already differentiated cells. Thus, by producing too much helper signal early in the inductive phase of the immune response, one can generate so much suppressor activity that one can abate the immune response almost totally; whereas, in the absence of this helper signal, either coming from T or B cells, the immune response would mature to a certain level before shutting itself off. This mechanism may be thought of as the "too-much-too-soon" hypothesis. It has long been known that antibody acts, through feedback, as an immunosuppressive agent. It is quite likely that one of the ways it acts in this fashion is via the "too-much-too-soon" mechanism. However, other mechanisms also play a role. These include diversion of antigen from the immune apparatus to the reticulo-endothelial system (predominantly in the liver), preventing antigen from being stimulatory; this is called the afferent suppression mechanism. In addition, there probably is an element of efferent suppression in which blocking antibodies, attached to targets of the immune system, block the activity of more potent humoral and cell-mediated immune mechanisms from reaching these targets and eliminating them.

(5) Miscellaneous

Undoubtedly other important mechanisms will be identified and expanded upon as new technological breakthroughs are achieved, but the four mechanisms mentioned above are presently the most important, well-identified ones. There are four other important, interesting new developments in the area of immuno-regulation which we would like to briefly mention here. Their precise role in regulating the immune response has not fully been worked out at this time, but it is apparent from the activity and interest in these areas that important, new information will soon be forthcoming. Recent reviews have appeared on these subjects to which the interested reader can refer for more detail.

Idiotype recognition (see 10, 11) An idiotype can be defined as that portion of an immunoglobulin molecule which gives the molecule antigen-recognizing capacity. The different amino acid sequences which endow antibody molecules with the ability to distinguish between antigens also gives them different antigenic characteristics, and these individual antigenic characteristics are refered to as idiotypes. Idiotype-anti-idiotype interactions between subsets of cells and humoral antibodies recently have been shown to both enhance and suppress specific portions of the immune response.

Allotype suppression (see 12) Allotypes are antigenic determinates on immunoglobulin molecules which are allelically expressed (like the Ly antigens), and not found on the hyper-variable portion of the molecule. The GM and INV systems in humans are examples of allotypes. In at least one mouse strain it has been shown that helper T cells seem to recognize allotypes on B cells and cooperate with the B cells via that allotypic recognition; and that suppressor T cells recognize something on the T cell which recognize the B cell allotype, and are able to suppress them via that recognition mechanism. Although only one example of this type of allotype regulation has been found, it is probable that others will be forthcoming in the near future.

Ia antigens (see 13) The antigens of the major histocompatibility complex (MHC) of mice and men were classically defined using cytotoxic antisera. Recently the use of mixed lymphocyte reactions has uncovered another region in the MHC which standard typing antisera do not pick up. The former antigens have been called S.D. (serologically defined) and the latter L.D. (lymphocyte defined). In the mouse the genetic loci which code for these antigens have been well worked out and 2 major regions have been defined: the I region (which contains L.D. determinants) and K, D region (which contains S.D. determinants). In humans the separation is not as clear, but D region antigens may be analogous to the I region in the mice (L.D.) and A, B, C antigens analogous to mouse K.D. Antigens coded for in the K and D regions of mice are expressed on essentially all cells; however, only some lymphocytes have the Ia antigens, and these seem to be much more heterogenous than K and D antigens. Thus, in the very near future it is likely that subsets of both T and B cells will be further defined using antisera directed against I region-coded antigens. The I region has gained particular importance in that it also codes for a number of factors which mediate both help and suppression in the interaction between subsets of T cells and between T cells and B cells.

Regulation of immunoglobulin synthesis (see 14) The very interesting work of Waldmann and his associates has shown that in some human cases of acquired hypogammaglobulinenemia, patients possess T cells which are capable of suppressing the pokeweed mitogen-induced, non-specific production of immunoglobulin molecules *in vitro*. The B cells of these patients seem to have no inherent defects, while their T cells suppress not only their own B cells in the pokeweed mitogen response, but also the B cells of normal people. Furthermore, Blaese and his associates (15) have uncovered a similar phenomenon in experimental animals. They showed that chickens which were made agammaglobulinenemic by removal of the bursa of Fabricius, and then irradiated, developed T cells which were capable of producing agammaglobulinenemia in non-bursectomized chickens.

The relationship of these four phenomena to one another, and to immunoregulation in general, is not clear at the present time. An interweaving thread would tie them together if one were to assume that there were differentiation antigens on subsets of cells which other subsets of T cells recognized, and that interactions among these subsets took place via the recognition of these differentiation antigens. Thus, in all four cases mentioned above, a common lesion could be either the experimental or induced loss, or excessive expression of these differentiation antigens on the target cell which could cause the regulating T cell to act aberrantly, either to produce too much help or too much suppression. That this is not too wild a speculation is supported by the findings that in chronic GVH disease too much T cell activity is produced due to the recognition of lymphocyte-expressed antigens, and this results in severe immunodeficiency.

SPECIFICITY AND MECHANISMS THROUGH WHICH IMMUNOREGULATION IS EFFECTED

The other points that remain to be covered:

(1) What is the specificity of all these reactions in terms of the

immunizing or tolerizing antigen? The answer to this is that there are some reactions which are exquisitvely specific in that both suppression and/or help require the initial antigen to be present for stimulation (1). Here regulatory factors resulting either in suppression or help work only on target cells which in turn react with the specific antigen. In other cases, the regulatory factors lack specificity for the immunizing or tolerizing antigen (1). The way that the specific and non- specific factors interact is not at all clear and one can see the great difficulties presented to scientists trying to work out the role of all of these heterogenous products and cells in the overall regulation of the immune response.

(2) How many of these effects are mediated by soluble factors, how many are mediated by cell contact, and what role does the macrophage play as an intermediary in passing information from one cell to the other? Again, all the answers to these questions are not available at present. It is clear, however, that some soluble factors are released into the supernatant after a T cell meets antigen, and that these factors appear to be of both specific and non-specific nature. It is also clear that not all the regulatory T cell effects can be accounted for by the soluble factors so far discovered, suggesting that cell-cell contact may also be playing an important role in immunoregulation (16).

Lastly, unpublished evidence from our laboratory indicates that the same can be said for the role of the macrophage as an intermediary. We have found that some, but not all, T-T and T-B interactions take place at the level of the macrophage membrane. We think that it is likely that the macrophage membrane is the site where interactions mediated by soluble factors are taking place, as we can block these interactions using factors which eliminate Fc receptor activity, but we can not affect the interactions by other treatments which do not affect Fc receptor activity.

REFERENCES

1. Gershon, R.K. 1974. In: Contemporary Topics in Immunobiology. 3: 1.

2. Scher, I., A.D. Steinberg, A.K. Berning and W.E. Paul. 1975. J. Exp. Med. 142: 637.

3. Andersson, B., and H. Blomgren. 1976. In: Immune Reactivity of Lymphocytes Development, Expression and Control. p. 283.

4. Raff, M.C., and H. Cantor. 1971. In: Progress in Immunology. p. 83.

5. Cantor, H., and E.A. Boyse. 1975. J. Exp. Med. 141: 1376.

6. Cantor, H., and E.A. Boyse. 1975. J. Exp. Med. 141: 1390.

7. Marchesi, V.T., and J.L. Gowans. 1964. Proc. Roy. Soc. Long. B. Biol. Sci. 159: 283.

8. Gershon, R.K. 1975. Transpl. Rev. 26: 170.

9. Gershon, R.K., Orbach-Arbouys, S., and C. Calkins. 1974. Prog. Immunol. II. 2: 123.

10. Eichmann, K., and K. Rajewsky. 1976. In: Cont. Topics in Immunobiol. 7 in press.

11. Wigzell, H., and H. Binz. 1976. In: Cont. Topics in Immunobiol. 7 in press.

12. Herzenberg, L.A., Okumura, K., and C.M. Metzler. 1975. Transpl. Rev. 27: 57.

13. Shreffler, D.C., and C.S. David. 1975. In: Advances in Immunology 20: 125.

14. Waldmann, T.A., S. Broder, M. Durm, M. Blackman and B. Meade. 1975. In: Immune Depression and Cancer. p. 20.

15. Blaese, R.M., Weiden, P.L., I. Koski, and N. Dooley. 1974. J. Exp. Med. 140: 1097.

16. Tadakuma, T., and C.W. Pierce. 1976. J. Exp. Med. in press.

IMMUNE COMPLEX DiSEASE

Charles G. Cochrane, M.D.

Department of Immunopathology, Scripps Clinic

La Jolla, California 92037

SUMMARY

Various types of injury induced by complexes of antigen and antibody are reviewed. These include reactions in which antibody reacts with antigens that are fixed in tissues or are soluble but localized at a particular site and reactions that occur following localization of circulating immunologic complexes in a particular tissue from the blood stream. Examples of each are reviewed.

The role of mediation systems in the pathogenesis of immunologic disease is stressed. Two examples of mediation pathways are provided in which a sequence of interacting humoral and cellular reactants is activated by antigen-antibody complex and which is responsible for the injurious consequences.

INTRODUCTION

Immunologic Mechanisms in Immune Complex Disease

The concept that antigen-antibody complex might cause disease was first suggested more than 60 years ago. In the course of studying serum sickness in humans, it was postulated that the coexistence of foreign serum antigens and homologous antibodies in the circulation resulted in the formation of toxic compounds which were probably the cause of the characterisitc lesions of this disease (1). Recently, much information has accumulated establishing the role of antigen-antibody complexes as pathogenetic agents capable of interacting with serum factors and/or cells to produce a variety of inflammatory and degenerative changes.

One of the principle findings that inititated recent studies on the relationship of immune complexes to disease was the observation that the lesions of serum sickness developed at the time of antigen-antibody interaction in the circulation (2,3). The earlier studies of anaphylaxis were extended to demonstrate that purified, soluble antigen-antibody complexes could, by themselves, induce systemic anaphylaxis (4). Also, it was shown that soluble antigen-antibody complexes would induce smooth muscle contraction in vitro (5), produce cutaneous reactions of increased vascular permeability (6), and even actual vascular necrosis (7). The study of experimental serum sickness employing isotopically labelled antigens and the fluorescent antibody technique demonstrated soluble, circulating antigen-antibody complexes during the development of the disease (8), and localization of antigen host Ig and host complement, presumably as immunologic complexes, in the lesion simulatenously with their development (9).

A partial definition of these properties of complex responsible for their pathogeneicity has been obtained. Germuth and McKinnon showed that complexes formed in moderate antigen excess, that is, complexes which were small enough to be soluble but were also capable of reacting with complement, were most active in producing systemic anaphylaxis (4).

The immunopathologic and clinical consequences of the presence of antigen-antibody complexes can vary greatly depending upon the anatomical sites of union of antigen and antibody and upon the absolute and relative amounts of the two reactants. In a broad sense there are three possible sites of antigen-antibody interaction and immune complex formation:

1. Injury produced by reaction of antibodies with structural antigens in tissues. When structural antigens making up part of the surface of cells or fixed intercellular structures react with antibody the immune complexes are essentially fixed at the site of the structural antigen and whatever inflammation or disease results from such

complexes is localized to a very specific site. The experimental disease nephrotoxic serum nephritis is an example of such immune complexes formed by passively transferred anti-GBM antibody which reacts with antigens of the GBM. Goodpasture's syndrome of man is a spontaneously occuring clinical disease similarly involving complexes of anti-basement membrane antibodies formed by the patient and structural basement membrane antigens.

The immunologic mechanisms in nephrotoxic nephritis illustrate this form of injury. When renal glomerular basement membrane (GBM) of one species is injected into a second species of animals, antibodies are formed which, when infused intravenously into the first, or donor, species bind along the GBM and induce glomerulonephritis. Disease results either from the initial reaction of heterologous antibody with donor GBM, or 8-10 days later, from the reaction of host antibodies directed against the GBM-bound heterologous immunoglobulin. Using immunofluorescent techniques, the immunoreactants can be readily observed at the site of injury: the

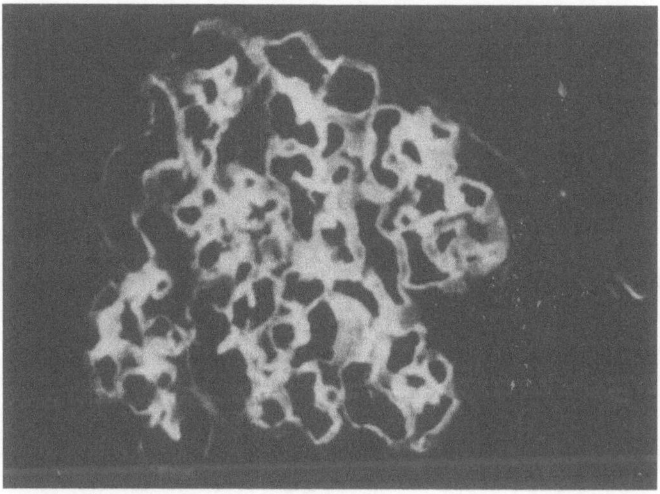

FIGURE 1

Fluorescent antibody localized anti-GBM antibody

heterologous immunoglobulin (Ig) and when present, the host Ig reacting against the GBM-bound, heterologous Ig, and complement components of the host reacting at the site. These features are illustrated in Figure 1.

Within a few hours after injection of antibodies to a recipient GBM, polymorphonuclear leukocytes (neutrophils) enter the reaction, force endothelial cells aside and gain intimate access to the complement and Ig on the surface of the GBM. This remarkable phenomenon is illustrated in Figures 2 and 3. It is at this time that proteinuria frequently makes its appearance. Within 6-12 hours, the neutrophils, leave the reaction site, leaving behind a severely damaged GBM structure.

This early injury is greatly augmented when the host produces Ig to the heterologous Ig. The newly-formed antibody then reacts with the remaining heterologous Ig bound to the GBM. At this time epithelial crescents form, and the glomeruli undergo permanent

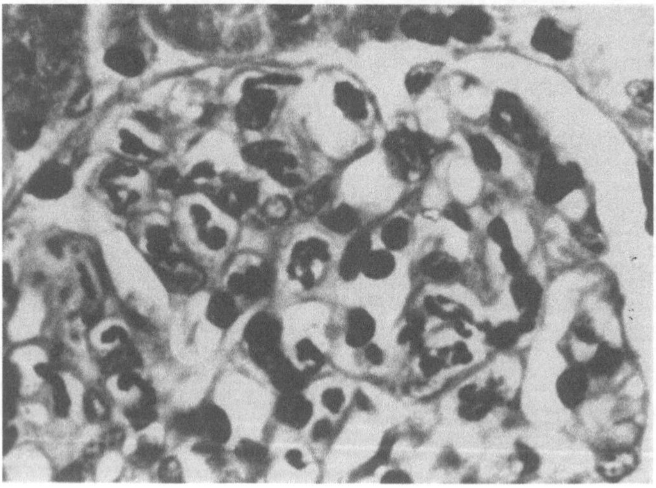

FIGURE 2

Neutrophil accumulation in anti-GBM nephritis

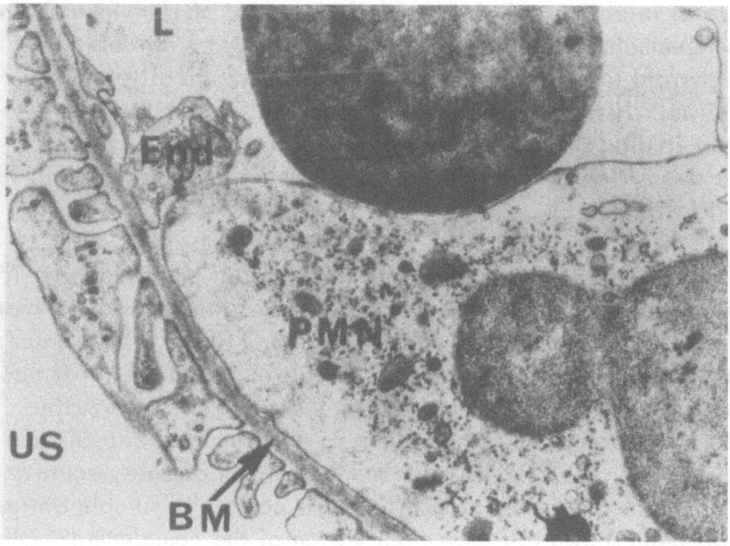

FIGURE 3

Electron microscopy of neutrophil in contact with GBM: L= lumen, End= endothelium, PMN= polymorphonuclear leukocyte, BM= basement membrane

sclerosis. The animal becomes uremic and undergoes progressive renal failure and eventual death. Greater detail of the immunologic events in this form of injury appears in a comphrehensive review by Unanue and Dixon (10).

2. Injury produced by reaction of antibodies with soluble antigen in tissues. When secreted or locally injected soluble antigens react with antibodies in sites very close to their point of origin the pathologic consequences of the formation of these localized soluble immune complexes tend to be similarly localized although not as sharply as in the case where the antigens are structurally fixed. The classical experimental example of this form of immune complex is the Arthus reaction wherein antigen injected in an intradermal site reacts with antibody in and about the blood vessels which carry the antibody to

the site of injection. A similar kind of deposit of complexes is found around spermatogenic tubules following vasectomy in rabbits and about thyroid follicles in animals with immunologically induced thyroiditis. Human thyroiditis, in which antibodies to thyroid hormones including thyroglobulin are formed spontaneously, has a similar deposition of localized soluble immune complexes about the thyroid follicles.

The Arthus reaction exemplifies this type of phenomenon. The Arthus reaction may be properly considered as the reaction in tissue produced by the complexing of antigen and antibody which causes the activation and local binding of complement and the focal accumulation of neutrophils. The mediating mechanisms of the Arthus reaction are common to many lesions of experimental animals and human beings. The arteritis of immune complex disease, acute nephrotoxic nephritis and immunologic synovitis caused by soluble antigens have all been shown to require activation of the complement system and accumulation of neutrophils as in the cutaneous Arthus reaction. In rheumatoid arthritis, acute glomerulonephritis, arteritis, acute homograft rejection and in other lesions as well, the hallmarks of the Arthus reaction have led investigators to an understanding of an underlying pathogenic mechanism.

Most commonly, the Arthus reaction is produced in experimental animals by the injection of antigen into the skin of a previously immunized animal with circulating precipitating antibody. A similar reaction develops when antibody is injected intradermally in an animal with circulating antigen. In either case, the immunologic reactants precipitate in the walls of venules within 15 minutes to an hour, and plasma complement is rapidly activated and bound. Neutrophils then enter the reaction over a period of 1-4 hours and severe injury of the vascular structures follows (Figure 4). More comprehensive accounting of this reaction is available in recent reviews (11,12).

3. Injury produced by the deposition of soluble immune complexes from the circulation into tissues. When soluble antigens are present in the circulation they react with antibodies and circulating immune complexes are formed; the size and solubility of which depend upon the ratios and amounts of antigen and antibody present and also upon

the size of the antigen. Such complexes may be trapped in one or more of the vascular or filtering structures of the body apparently for anatomical and physiological reasons. Such complexes are without immunologic relationship to their sites of deposit and therefore the tissues injured are truly innocent bystanders in contrast to the direct antigenic involvement of the tissues in the first two forms of immune complex disease. The classical experimental model of systemic immune complex disease is serum sickness in which kidneys, heart, blood vessels, lungs, spleen, joints and choroid plexus all may be involved by deposition of immune complexes with subsequent phlogogenic changes. In clinical medicine primary immune complex diseases include lupus erythematosus, most glomerulonephritides, a variety of vasculitides and rheumatoid arthritis. In addition, both acute and chronic infections and infestations usually give rise to circulating immune complexes which may contribute significantly to the injury associated with these diseases.

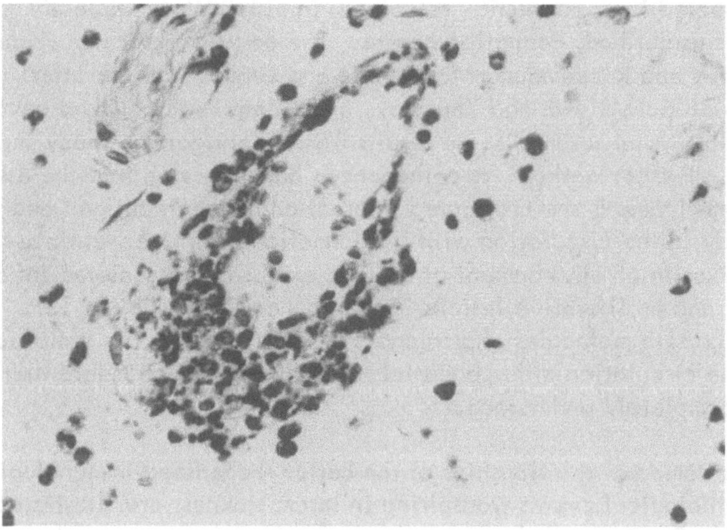

FIGURE 4

Localized Arthus reaction

Experimental serum sickness is of considerable interest for several reasons. First, it corresponds closely to clinical serum sickness, a not uncommon iatrogenic complication of serum therapy, and has provided a useful model for the study of this disease. Second, the signs, symptoms, and morphological lesions of serum sickness bear close resemblance to some of the changes seen in various poorly understood human diseases of the connective tissues and certain drug reactions. Third, the pathogenic mechanisms which have been defined in studies of experimental serum sickness also may be operative in those clinical diseases which it resembles: rheumatoid arthritis, rheumatic fever, disseminated lupus erythematosus, glomerulonephritis, polyarteritis, and certain purpuras.

Experimental acute serum sickness is produced by one or several closely spaced, relatively large injections of heterologous serum protein into an animal with little or no preexisiting homologous antibody. In the case of the initial exposure to a given foreign protein, there is no preexisiting antibody and the disease develops one to two weeks after injection; if it is a repeated exposure, some preexisiting antibody may be present and the disease develops sooner, as would be expected in an amanestic response. In either case, disease appears as antibody formation begins. The early work of von Priquet, Longcope and Rackemann, MacKenzie and Leake, and the later studies of Rich, Hawn and Janeway, and Germuth established beyond much doubt that serum disease results from an antigen-antibody interaction. Further work on its pathogenesis has suggested that the essence of serum sicness is the protracted interaction between antigen and antibody in the circulation with the formation of antigen-antibody complexes in an environment of antigen excess and associated inflammatory and proliferative lesions in the connective tissue (9, 13). Serum protein molecules, homologous or heterologous, are removed from the circulation at exponential rates by nonimmune means that are incompletely understood.

The temporal relationships of the better recognized immunological and pathological events transpiring in serum sickness are illustrated in Figure 5. Data for this figure were obtained from previously unimmunized rabbits given intravenous injections of 0.25 g of ^{131}I-labelled bovine serum albumin (I*BSA) per kilogram of body weight. Except for differences in the time of onset of the response, these observations

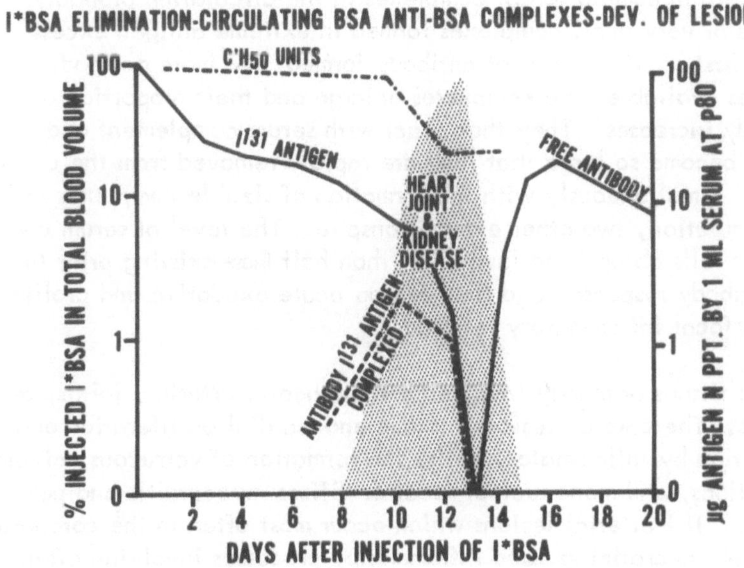

FIGURE 5

Elimination of I-BSA and production of serum sickness

apply to human or experimental serum sickness induced with a large dose of virtually any serum protein antigen. The solid line indicating the level of ^{131}I-antigen in the blood shows a rapid fall during the first two days as the intravenously injected antigen equilibrates between intra-and extra- vascular components of the serum protein pool. There follows a relatively slow, nonimmune decline lasting a little more than a week, and then the remaining antigen is rapidly eliminated from the circulation within two days. Following the elimination of circulating antigen, free antibody promptly appears in the serum. The rapid final elimination of circulating antigen is caused by the production of antibody which combines with circulating antigen, forming antigen-antibody complexes which are removed from the circulation. The amounts of detectable circulating complexes are indicated by the dotted line beginning about seven days after administration of antigen and increasing to a maximum at ten days, just prior to the beginning of rapid immune elimination of antigen.

The initial accumulation of complexes in the circulation probably consists of very small complexes formed in extreme antigen excess by the first small amounts of antibody formed. As more antibody becomes available, the complexes enlarge and their proportion of antibody increases. They then react with serum complement and finally become so large that they are rapidly removed from the circulation. Simultaneously with the formation of sizable complexes in the circulation, two other events transpire. The level of serum complement falls abruptly to levels less than half those existing prior to the antibody response, and they develop acute exudative and proliferative focal inflammatory lesions.

The tissues primarily involved are the heart, arteries, joints, and kidneys. The cardiac lesions include endocardial proliferation and infiltration by inflammatory cells, the formation of verrucous valvular vegetations, and mononuclear focal or diffuse myocarditis and pericarditis. The arterial lesions which occur most often in the coronaries are focal, necrotizing, and inflammatory processes involving often all layers of the arterial wall. The lesions may show an acute inflammatory exudate, necrosis of the arterial wall, and fibrinoid material or

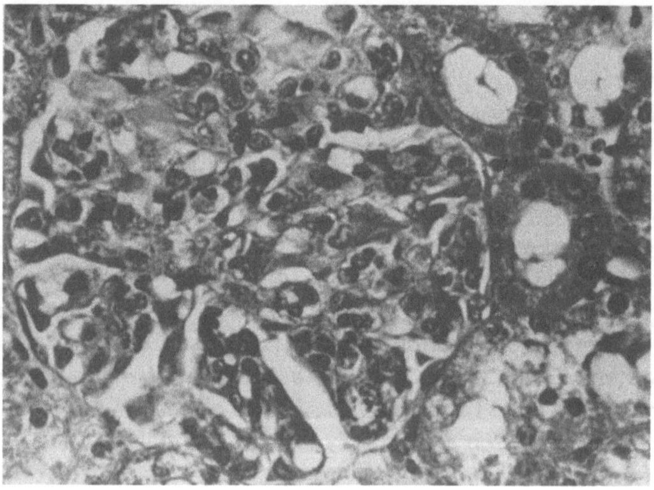

FIGURE 6

Serum sickness in the kidney

may be primarily a mononuclear reaction. The kidneys show extensive uniform endothelial proliferation of glomerular capillaries with slight basement membrane thickening (Figure 6). After the elimination of complexes from the circulation, the lesions rapidly disappear, and in most instances healing is complete.

By immunohistochemical techniques, antigen, host complement and host γ-globulin presumably in complex form, are found to localize specifically in tissue lesions simultaneously with their development (9) and thus appear to be etiological agents of tissue injury. Apparently the earliest phlogogenic stimulus initiating the focal inflammatory lesions in serum sickness results from an antigen-antibody interaction, causing systemic liberation of active pharmacological agents which increase vascular permeability (14). Following this, circulating complexes begin to accumulate in vessel walls, particularily in focal fashion, along the internal elastic lamina of arteries and the basement membranes of glomeruli. Next, after complement activation by the complexes, polymorphonuclear leukocytes accumulate at sites of complex deposition in arteries and produce considerable vascular damage and necrosis.

If antigen-antibody complexes are involved in the chronic clinical diseases mentioned above, it seems likely that experimental conditions designed to keep small amounts of such complexes present in the circulation for long periods of time should produce chronic progressive disease. Dixon and his colleagues extended earlier efforts to make such a model (15), injecting intravenously small amounts of heterologous serum proteins daily into rabbits (16). Bovine serum albumin, human serum albumin, bovine γ-globulin, and human γ-globulin all served as satisfactory antigens. The antibody responses to daily injection of these antigens varied, and it was animals producing moderate amounts that were most prone to disease. These animals formed soluble antigen-antibody complexes which persisted in the circulation for much of the interval between the daily antigen injections.

The chronic glomerulonephritis was detectable clinically by proteinuria, in some instances hematuria, hypoproteinemia, and elevated serum cholesterol and urea levels. The most common and probably the earliest anatomic form of this disease was a membranous glomerulonephritis characterized by thickened glomerular capillary basement

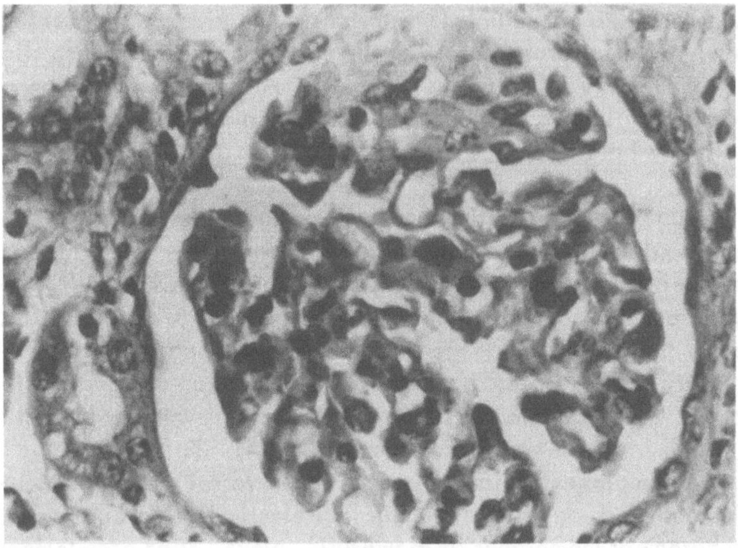

FIGURE 7

Chronic glomerulonephritis

membranes with little or no endothelial proliferation (Figure 7). This lesion was much less inflammatory than degenerative by morphologic criteria. As the disease progressed, proliferative and scarring reactions became more evident. Again, as would be expected if the complexes were causing this renal lesion, antigen, host γ-globulin and host complement were found concentrated in the thickened basement membranes (Figure 8). By electron microscopy a lumpy, dense deposit was seen along the outer aspect of the basement membranes corresponding to the antigen, γ -globulin, and complement-rich deposits visualized with the fluorescent antibody technique (Figure 9). Subsequent electron microscopic studies with ferritin-labelled antibody have confirmed this correspondence (14). Once in this site, the immunologic reactants and the morphologically demonstrable deposits persisted for long periods--as much as one year after cessation of antigen injections--with persistence of associated renal malfunction.

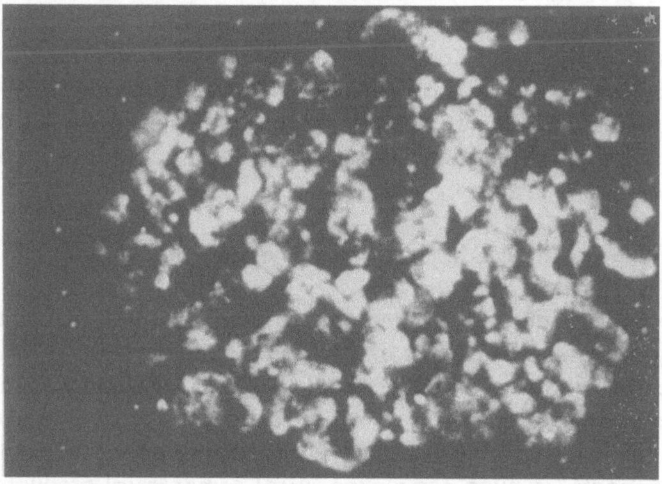

FIGURE 8

Fluorescent antibody localized immune complex mediated glomerulonephritis

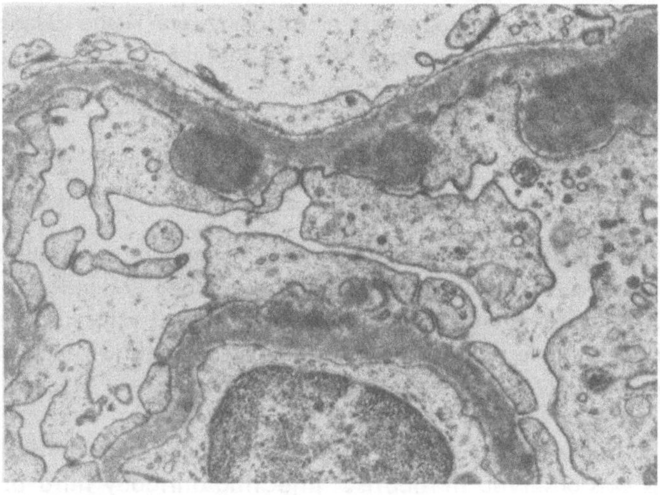

FIGURE 9

Electron microscopic observation of immune complex deposition

In the prolonged daily exposure to low levels of circulating complexes, the kidneys were the only organs injured. When large amounts of antigen were administered to rabbits producing considerable antibody, deposits of immune complexes appeared in the alveolar walls and interstitium of the lung. Pneumonitis resulted, marked by fibrin deposition, inflammatory cell accumulation and fibrosis (17).

The Mediation of Immune Complex Injury

An understanding of immunologic disease involves knowledge of not only inciting agents, but of mediation systems as well. With evidence at hand that an understanding of inciting agents (viruses, etc.) is extremely complex, it behooves investigators to examine the mechanisms by which host mediatory systems are activated by the inciting agents (immune complexes, viral or bacterial products, etc.) and how they cause injury to the tissues. Through an analysis of these humoral and cellular systems rational therapeutic means may be devised to block the reaction sequences from progressing to the point of structural injury of tissues.

Two reaction sequences will be used to illustrate the role of mediation systems in the pathogenesis of inflammatory tissue damage. It will become apparent that many links in the chain of events are susceptible to therapeutic intervention.

1. Immunologic injury mediated by polymorphonuclear leukocytes and complement.

a. A role of PMN's in tissue injury. The Arthus vasculitis is the first antigen-antibody induced lesion to be found dependent upon PMN's. Specific removal of PMN's by treatment with nitrogen mustard or heterologous anti-PMN sera has been shown to lead to striking inhibition of the reaction in several species (18-21).

A similar dependence upon PMN's of immunologically induced synovitis was observed in rabbits. Injecting antibody intra-articularly in rabbits with circulating antigen induced a severe synovitis that was markedly inhibited by PMN depletion (22). Of special interest, it was found possible to re-establish synovial injury in a PMN depleted rabbit by infusing a suspension of freshly isolated PMN's obtained from the peripheral circulation of normal rabbits (23). Such a reconstitution of injury substantiated the hypothesis that PMN's play an important role in the mediation of vascular injury by antigen-antibody complexes.

In serum sickness of rabbits, when PMN's were removed just prior to development of the lesions, the usual necrotizing arteritis did not appear. Intimal proliferation was markedly inhibited or absent, PMN infiltration did not occur, and there was not destruction of the internal elastic lamina or fibrinoid necrosis in the arterial walls (24). The glomerulitis, normally seen in serum sickness, was not affected by PMN removal. This was not surprising in view of the paucity of PMN's in glomeruli in acute immune complex disease of rabbits.

In acute nephrotoxic nephritis, a disease based on the reaction of injected antibody with the glomerular basement membrane, a clear role of PMN's also was apparent in the development of injury. Within two hours after the injection of antibody, a large accumulation of PMN's was observed in the glomeruli (25). This accumulation lasted for about 6 hours and the numbers of PMN's found thereafter in the glomeruli diminished. Proteinuria was first detected when PMN's were accumulating and the numbers of PMN's in the glomeruli correlated well with the amount of protein in the urine. Removal of the PMN's by using either purified anti-PMN antibody or nitrogen mustard markedly or completely inhibited the occurence of proteinuria (Table 1). Depletion of PMN's failed to inhibit antibody and host complement binding in the glomeruli. As in the Arthus reaction, when large amounts of antibody were used, glomerular permeability increased in spite of the absence of PMN's. This indicated that factors other than those in PMN's could take part in the development of injury to the glomerulus. A similar immunologic permeability reaction is noted when antibodies to vascular basement membrane were injected intradermally. Both PMN-dependent and -independent reactions could be elicited in several species.

b. Mechanisms of accumulation of polymorphonuclear leukocytes: a role of complement. Present concepts as to the mechanisms of accumulation of PMN's are based solely on the multitudinous studies of this process in general inflammation. These studies have demonstrated

TABLE 1

PROTEINURIA IN FIRST 24 HOURS AFTER INJECTION

OF MODERATE DOSAGE OF NEPHROTOXIC SERUM

	Normal		PMN depleted	
	No.	mg/24 hours	No.	mg/24 hours
Rats	8	246		59
	6	50		6
Rabbits	5	1843		0.2

TABLE 2

EFFECT OF COMPLEMENT DEPLETION ON PMN ACCUMULATION

IN ARTHUS REACTION AND EARLY NEPHROTOXIC NEPHRITIS

	No. of Rats	PMN Accumulation	Fluorescent Results C'	Fluorescent Results AgAb	$C'H_{50}$	PMN (Per MM^3)	Platelets
Nephrotoxic nephritis							
C-depleted	7	-	±	4+	< 7.5	10,960	-
Controls	6	+	3+	4+	38	4,200	-
Arthus							
C-depleted	10	-	±	4	< 8	7,300	591,000
Controls	5	+	3+	4+	49	4,300	610,000

several important concepts, among which are: 1) A humoral factor may well exist in areas of inflammation capable of attracting PMN's into the site of injury. While early evidence was inconsistent with this (26) studies by Buckley employing micro foci of injury have been most indicative (27). 2) From in vitro studies there is some evidence suggesting a serum factor that may be important in the attraction of PMN's toward a site of tissue injury (28,29). From in vitro studies employing a wide variety of substances that are chemotactic, from washed bacteria to extracts of burned tissue and serum, it would appear that there may be more than one stubstance capable of attracting PMN's chemotactically.

Studies on the attraction of PMN's to immunologic reactants in tissues have strongly implicated plasma complement as being essential for the generation of the chemotactic factor. Four reactions have been studied in detail, the Arthus phenomenon (30), acute nephrotoxic nephritis (25), arteritis associated with immune complex deposition (24), and synovitis resulting from antigen-antibody combination in small vessels in joint tissues (22). Two approaches were taken, the first consisting of depleting animals of plasma complement prior to induction of reactions, and the second of using antibodies to induce reactions (in normal animals) that were incapable of fixing complement. Under both circumstances PMN infiltration was absent, even though antigen and antibody deposits were detected in the vessel walls with fluorescent antibody techniques. In each case, however, little or no C3 could be found in the vascular structure. Thus, in both C-depleted and normal animals, a correlation existed between the ability of the antibody to fix C and the accumulation of PMN's at the antigen-antibody site (Table 2).

Complement might bring about the accumulation of PMN in two ways: 1) Through immune adherence; and 2) By releasing chemotactic agents that cause a directional migration of PMN toward the point of greatest concentration, i.e. the antigen-antibody complex where complement components are being activated.

Immune adherence is a phenomenon by which PMN and macrophages from most species, platelets from some species and erythrocytes only of primates bind to an immune aggregate. In a few species the IgG antibody together with antigen is sufficient to induce adherence of the cells, but in all species the fixation of complement, especially the third component, greatly augments the adherence. Presumably, when immune complexes deposit or form in blood vessel walls and complement through the third component is bound, PMN in the circulation would bind. This would be eliminated by depletion of C3, as was accomplished in the experiments noted in Table 2. Until recently chemotaxis has been a phenomenon observed exclusively in vitro. The directional migration of PMN's to a source of a humoral stimulating agent has been successfully examined in chambers, separated into two compartments by a microport filter. Cells such as PMN, placed in the upper chamber, migrate through the filter to a source of chemotactic material in the bottom compartment. By this method, antigen-antibody complexes were observed to generate chemotactic activity from fresh serum with an intact complement system (31, 32). Subsequently, three chemotactic agents have been derived from activated components of complement, C5-6-7 complex (32, 33), $C3_a$ (34, 35), $C5_a$ (36, 37). Recently, a role of chemotaxis has been observed in vivo. In synovial tissues, PMN' s were observed to migrate over 200 microns to appoint where complement components were activated by an immunologic reaction (23). Blocking activation of the complement system inhibited migration of the PMN's.

Thus complement appears to play an important role in the accumulation of PMN's at the site of immunologic reactions.

c. The role of PMN leukocytic proteases and basic peptides in the alteration of vascular integrity. In further considerations of the apparent attack of PMN's on basement membranes, it was found that lysates of PMN's or the PMN cytoplasmic granules were capable of attacking semipurified glomerular basement membrane in vitro (38). These studies showed that peptides were released from the basement membrane by the PMN lysates. The agents responsible were found to be cathepsins D and E of rabbit PMN's (38).

In human PMN's a neutral protease will hydrolyze isolated basement membrane much in the same way as the acid cathepsins of rabbit PMN's (39). PMN's also contain a collagenase that attacks basement membranes (40, 41). In addition, an elastase has been isolated that cleaves porcine elastin (40). This may be the enzyme responsible for breakdown of the internal elastic lamina of arteries observed in serum sickness (24).

At least four basic proteins have been isolated from the lysosomes of PMN that are capable of increasing vascular permeability. The effect of one of these follows its action on most cells and the consequent release of histamine (42). The other three act independently by means as yet unclear (43).

A composite of the numerous potential agents by which PMN can mediate injury of vessels is shown in Table 3. The relationship of these mediating factors in the pathogenesis of several disease models is given in Figure 10.

TABLE 3

POTENTIALLY INJURIOUS CONSTITUENTS OF PMN

Acid phosphatase	
Lysozyme	
Collagenase	
Aryl sulfatases	
Acid lipase	
Endogenous pyrogen	
Basic proteins:	(a) Mast-cell-active
	(b) Permeability-inducing, independent of mast cells
Elastase	
Neutral protease	
Acid protease (cathepsins)	
Fibrinolysin	
Procoagulant:	(a) Tissue factor
	(b) Precipitation of fibrin monomers and anti-heparin effect by basic proteins
Mononuclear cell chemotactic factor	
Oxidizing substances--superoxides, singlet oxygen, hydrogen peroxide	

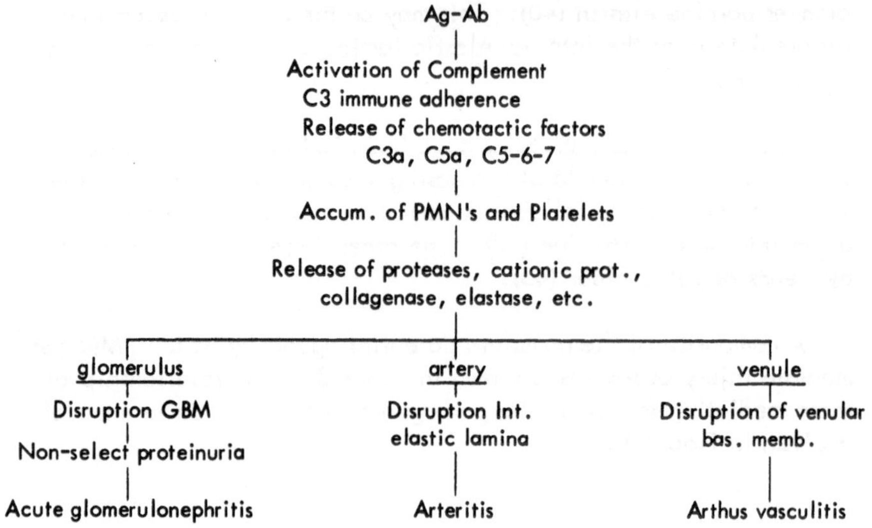

FIGURE 10

Pathogenesis of immune complex disease

2. Mediation systems responsible for the deposition in tissues of circulating immune complexes.

In serum sickness as noted above, the experimental evidence has indicated that the lesions result from the localization of circulating immune complexes. The means by which the circulating complexes localize in vessel walls apparently involves the participation of an anaphylactic triggering mechanism. This mechanism illustrates a second pathway involving several interacting host factors.

Studies to date (44,45) of the physiochemical properties of circulating soluble antigen-antibody complexes that govern their ability to to localize in vessles subjected to increased permeability have indicated that: 1) increased permeability of the vessel is necessary for localization to occur; 2) there is no detectable affinity of soluble complexes for the basement membrane or "activated" endothelial cells;

and 3) the complexes and other macromolecules apparently localized because of their large size, i.e., they are trapped along the basement membrane filter.

Further studies of acute immune complex disease in rabbits have suggested that similar mechanisms may be involved in the localization of circulating immune complexes. Carbon injected intravenously to serve as a marker during the onset of serum sickness was found to localize along the internal elastic lamina of large arteries in the early lesion sites (14). When antagonists of vasoactive amines were administered in high doses just prior to development of the disease, complexes failed to localize and the lesions were largely inhibited. Depletion of the major source of vasoactive amines in the blood of rabbits, i.e., the platelets, had a similar effect. The treatment did not inhibit the formation and production of complexes. Surprisingly, glomerular localization of the complexes, glomerular lesions, and proteinuria were also diminished by both antihistamine-antiserotonin treatment and platelet depletion. These data contrasted with the expectation that circulating complexes would localize on the glomerular basement membrane owing to the natural filtration already existing in the glomerulus. In the presence of vasoactive amines, a contributing factor influencing the localization of complexes in serum sickness was apparently the turbulence of flow (14).

The size of the circulating immune complexes is also important in determining whether deposition of the complexes and development of lesions occur. In a correlative study, deposition of circulating complexes and development of glomerular and arterial lesions in acute immune complex disease of rabbits were found almost exclusively in animals forming large complexes, i.e., greater than 19 x in size (46). In chronic immune complex disease in rabbits, a similar correlation between large complexes in the circulation and deposition in glomeruli was observed (47).

It is clear from the above observations, that a trigger mechanism of increasing vascular permeability plays a role in the deposition of large circulating complexes in vessel walls and along the glomerular basement membrane. The increased vascular permeability depends in some way upon platelets and, apparently, their content of vasoactive amines. Analyses of the interaction of immune complexes and

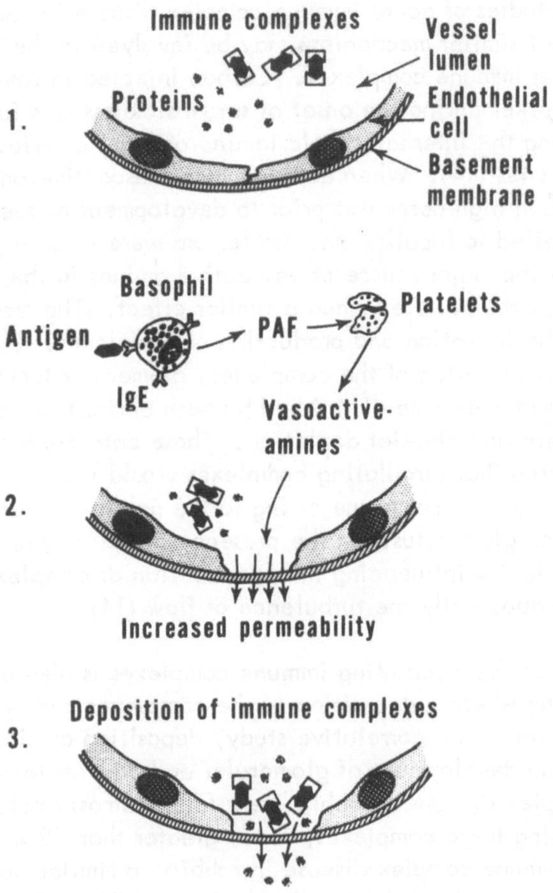

FIGURE 11

Proposed mechanism of immune complex disease

platelets of rabbits have revealed three mechanisms by which the platelets released their histamine and serotonin, each requiring complement (for review, see 48). In addition, a fourth mechanism has been studied by which basophils of sensitized rabbits, on contact with antigen and in the absence of complement, evidence of clumping of platelets and release of the vasoactive amines (48). A soluble, low molecular weight (1200 daltons) factor has been described, entitled platelet activating factor (PAF) which is released from IgE sensitized basophils and induces clumping and release of vasoactive amines from platelets (49). The complement-dependent mechanisms were found not to play a significant role in the deposition of circulating complexes. Rabbits, depleted of C3 and terminal components of complement still developed glomerulitis and arteritis of acute immune complex disease with attendant deposition of the complexes in lesions (50). By contrast, the presence of the basophil-dependent mechanism correlated well with the deposition of complexes and development of glomerulonephritis and arteritis. Evidence therefore suggested that basophils from sensitized rabbits react with antigen in the circulation to bring about an anaphylactic reaction that incorporates the participation of platelets. The platelets then, possibly by releasing vasoactive amines, increase local vascular permeability allowing macromolecular complexes in the circulation to deposit circulating complexes in glomeruli and blood vessels to initiate immune complex disease (Figure II).

REFERENCES

1. Von Pirquet, C.E.: Allergy. Arch. Intern. Med. 7: 259, 1911.

2. Hawn, C.V.Z. and Janeway, C.A.: Histologic and serological sequences in experimental hypersensitivity. J. Exp. Med. 85: 571, 1947.

3. Germuth, F. G.: A comparative histologic and immunologic study in rabbits of induced hypersensitivity of the serum sickness type. J. Exp. Med. 97: 257, 1953.

4. Germuth, F.G., and McKinnon, G.E.: Studies on the biological properties of antigen-antibody complexes. I. Anaphylactic shock induced by soluble antigen-antibody complexes in unsensitized normal guinea pigs. Bull. Johns Hopkins Hosp. 101: 13, 1957.

5. Trapani, I.L., Garvey, J.S. and Campbell, D.: Stimulating action of soluble antigen-antibody complexes on normal guinea pig smooth muscle. Science 127: 700, 1958.

6. Ishizaka, K., and Campbell, D.H.: Biological activity of soluble antigen-antibody complexes. I. Skin reactive properties. Proc. Soc. Exp. Biol. Med. 97: 635, 1958.

7. Cochrane, C.G., and Weigle, W.O.: The cutaneous reaction to soluble antigen antibody complexes. A comparison with the Arthus phenomenon. J. Exp. Med. 108: 591, 1957.

8. Dixon, F.J.: Characterization of the antibody response. J. Cell. Comp. Physiol. 50: 27, 1957.

9. Dixon, F.J., Vazquez, J.J., Weigle, W.O., and Cochrane, C.G.: Pathogenesis of serum sickness. Arch. Path. 65: 18, 1958.

10. Unanue, E.R. and Dixon, F.J.: Experimental glomerulonephritis: Immunological events and pathogenetic mechanisms. Adv. in Immunol. 6: 1, 1967.

11. Cochrane, C.G.: Immunologic tissue injury mediated by neutrophilic leukocytes. Adv. In Immunol. 9: 97, 1968.

12. Cochrane, C.G., and Janoff, A.: The Aruthus reaction: A model of neutrophil and complement mediated injury. In: The Inflammatory Process, Vo. 3, pp. 85-162, 1974.

13. Dixon, F.J.: The role of antigen-antibody complexes in disease. Harvey Lect. 58: 21, 1963.

14. Andres, G.A., Seegal, B.C., Hsu, K.C., Rothenberg, M.S. and Chapeau, M.L.: Electron microscopic studies of experimental nephritis with ferritin-conjugated antibody. Localization of antigen-antibody complexes in rabbit glomeruli following repeated injections of bovine serum albumin. J. Exp. Med. 117: 691, 1963.

15. McLean, C.R., Fitzgerald, J.D.L., Younghusband, O.Z. and Hamilton, J.D.: Diffuse glomerulonephritis induced in rabbits by small intravenous injections of horse serum. Arch. Path. 51: 1, 1951.

16. Dixon, F.J., Feldman, J.D., and Vazquez, J.J.: Experimental glomerulonephritis. The pathogenesis of a laboratory model resembling the spectrum of human glomerulonephritis. J. Exp. Med. 113: 899, 1961.

17. Bentjens, J.R., O'Connell, D.W., Pawlowski, J.B., Hsu, K.C., and Andres, G.A.: Experimental immune complex disease of the lung. The pathogenesis of a laboratory model resembling certain human interstitial lung disease. J. Exp. Med. 140: 105, 1974.

18. Cochrane, C.G., Weigle, W.O., and Dixon, F.J.: The role of polymorphonuclear leukocytes in the initiation and cessation of the Arthus vasculitis. J. Exp. Med. 110: 481, 1959.

19. Humphrey, J.H.: The mechanism of the Arthus reactions. I. The role of polymorphonuclear leukocytes and platelets in reversed passive Arthus reactions in rabbits. Brit. J. Exp. Path. 36: 268, 1955.

20. Humphrey, J.H.: The mechanism of the Arthus reactions. II. The role of polymorphonuclear leukocytes and platelets in reversed passive Arthus reactions in the guinea pig. Brit. J. Exp. Path. 36:

21. Stetson, C.A.: Similarities in the mechanisms determining the Arthus and Shwartzman phenomena. J.Exp. Med. 94: 347, 1951.

22. DeShazo, C.V., Henson, P. M., and Cochrane, C.G.: Acute immunologic arthritis in rabbits. J. Clin. Invest. 51: 50, 1972.

23. DeShazo, C.V., McGrade, M.T., Henson, P.M. and Cochrane, C.G.: The effect of complement depletion on neutrophil migration in acute immunologic nephritis. J. Immunol. 108: 1414, 1972.

24. Kniker, W.T., and Cochrane, C.G.: Pathogenetic factors in vascular lesions of experimental serum sickness. J. Exp. Med. 122: 83, 1965.

25. Cochrane, C.G., Unanue, E.R., and Dixon, F.J.: A role of polymorphonuclear leukocytes and complement in nephrotoxic nephritis. J. Exp. Med. 122: 99, 1965.

26. Harris, H.: Role of chemotaxis in inflammation. Physiol. Rev. 34: 529, 1954.

27. Buckley, I.K.: Delayed secondary damage and leukocyte chemotaxis following focal aseptic heat injury in vivo. Exp. Molec. Path. 2: 402, 1963.

28. Hurley, J.V.: Substances promoting luekocyte emigration. In: The Acute Inflammatory Process. N.Y. Acad. Sci.116: 918, 1964.

29. Hurley, J.V., and Spector, W.G.: Endogenous factors responsible for leukocyte emigration in vivo. J. Path. Bact. 82: 403, 1961.

30. Ward, P.A., and Cochrane, C.G.: Bound complement and immunologic injury of blood vessels. J. Exp. Med. 121: 215, 1965.

31. Boyden, S.: The chemotactic effect of mixtures of antibody and antigen on polymorphonuclear leukocytes. J. Exp. Med. 115: 453, 1962.

32. Ward, P.A., Cochrane, C.G., and Muller-Eberhard, H.J.: The role of serum complement in chemotaxis of leukocytes in vitro. J. Exp. Med. 122: 327, 1965.

33. Ward, P.A., Cochrane, C.G., and Muller-Eberhard, H.J.: Further studies on the chemotactic factor of complement and its formation in vivo. Immunol. 11: 141, 1966.

34. Bokisch, V.A., Muller-Eberhard, H.J., and Cochrane, C.G.: Isolation of a fragment (C3a) of the third component of human complement containing anaphylatoxin and chemotactic activity and description of an anaphylatoxin inactivator of human serum. J. Exp. Med. 129: 1109, 1969.

35. Ward, P.A.: A plasmin-split fragment of C'3' as a new chemotactic facotr. J. Exp. Med. 126: 189, 1967.

36. Shin, H.S., Pickering, R.J., Mayer, M.M., and Cook, C.T.: Guinea pig C'5'. J. Immunol. 101: 813 (abstract), 1968.

37. Ward, P.A., and Newman, L.J.: A neutrophil chemotactic factor from C'5'. J. Immunol. 102: 93, 1969.

38. Cochrane, C.G., and Aikin, B.S.: Polymorphonuclear leukocytes in immunologic reactions. The destruction of vascular basement membrane in vivo and in vitro. J. Exp. Med. 124: 733, 1966.

39. Janoff, A., and Zeligs, J.D.: Vascular injury and lysis of basement membrane in vitro by neutral protease of human leukocytes. Science 161: 702, 1968.

40. Janoff, A., and Sherer, J.: Mediators of inflammation in leukocyte lysosomes. IX. Elastinolytic activity in granules of human polymorphonuclear leukocytes. J. Exp. Med. 128: 1137, 1968.

41. Lazarus, G.S., Brown, R.S., Daniels, J.R., and Fullmer, H.M. H.M.: Human granulocyte collagenase. Science 159: 1483, 1968.

42. Janoff, A., Schaeffer, S., Scherer, J., and Bran, M.A.: Mediators of inflammation in leukocyte lysosomes. II. Mechanism of action of lysosomal cationic protein upon vascular permeability in the rat. J. Exp. Med. 128: 841, 1965.

43. Randadive, N.S., and Cochrane, C.G.: Isolation and characterization of permeability factors from rabbit neutrophils. J. Exp. Med. 128: 605, 1968.

44. Cochrane, C.G.: Studies on the localization of circulating antigen-antibody complexes and other macromolecules in vessels. I. Structural studies. J. Exp. Med. 118: 489, 1963.

45. Cochrane, C.G.: Studies on the localization of circulating antigen-antibody complexes and other macromolecules in vessels. II. Pathogeneic and pharmacodynamic studies. J. Exp. Med. 118: 503, 1963.

46. Cochrane, C.G., and Hawkins, D.: Studies on circulating immune complexes. III. Factors governing the ability of circulating complexes to localize in blood vessels. J. Exp. Med. 127: 137, 1968.

47. Wilson, C.B., and Dixon, F.J.: Quantitation of acute and chronic serum sickness in the rabbit. J. Exp. Med. 134: 7s, 1971.

48. Cochrane, C.G., and Koffler, D.: Immune complex disease in experimental animals and man. In: Advances in Immunology. F.J. Dixon and H.G. Kunkel, eds. Vol. 16. New York, Academic Press, Inc. pp. 185-264, 1973.

49. Benveniste, J., Henson, P.M., and Cochrane, C.G.: Leucocyte-dependent histamine release from rabbit platelets. The role of IgE, basophils and a platelet-activating factor. J. Exp. Med. 136: 1356, 1972.

50. Ishizaka, K., and Campbell, D.H.: Biologic activity of soluble antigen-antibody complexes. IV. The inhibition of the skin reacitivy of soluble complexes and the PCA reaction by heterologous complexes. J. Immunol. 83: 116, 1959.

THE ROLE OF CHRONIC VIRAL INFECTION IN IMMUNOLOGIC DISEASE

Frank J. Dixon, M.D.

Director, Scripps Clinic and Research Foundation
La Jolla, California 92037

We know a fair amount about how immunologic disease develops and how immunologic reactions trigger humoral and cellular mediators to produce tissue injury. This knowledge has accumulated over the past two decades largely because of the technological and conceptual developments in the field of immunology. These developments have allowed us, first, to quantitate the very basic elements of immunologic reactions: the presence and class of immunoglobulin molecules, the components of complement, and the various kinds of lymphocytes and, second, to determine in which disease states abnormalities of these elements occur. We have been able to link immunologic abnormalities with diseases that, 20 years ago, completely eluded our understanding. Present assays for immune complexes, for auto-antibodies and for abnormally reactive lymphocytes provide the results suggesting specific immunopathologic mechanisms at work in human diseases such as glomerulonephritis, rheumatoid arthritis, systemic lupus erythematosus, a variety of vasculidites, thyroiditis and many other endocrine abnormalities, hepatitis, myasthenia gravis and probably less clearly understood diseases such as multiple sclerosis and subacute sclerosing panencephalitis. In spite of this combination of very sophisticated immunologic information and suspicion, which is really what it is, we have very little understanding of etiologic agents in most of these diseases. It's one thing to analyze a disease like glomerulonephritis and say, "We know absolutely this is caused by immune complex deposits or by antibodies to glomerular basement membrane (GBM). In a renal biopsy we can see immune complexes or anti-GBM antibodies by using immunofluorescence. Eluting that renal biopsy, we can find the very antibodies that have injured the kidney." All that is fine. But we still don't know what has set the reaction in motion. Why do some people make antibodies against their basement membranes or circulating potential immunogens? Even though we know that antibodies exist, and we know exactly how disease develops once they are there, we don't know how their formation was initiated.

The studies I would like to talk about involve several attempts to evaluate the potential of chronic viral infections as prototype etiologic agents for various immunologic diseases, the causes of which are poorly understood. The question was, do chronic experimental viral infections, in certain situations, produce diseases that look like suspected immunologic diseases of man? The answer is yes, that a variety of chronic viral infections of animals do produce immunologic disease reminisicent of a number of human diseases.

First we will consider chronic viral infection and the kinds of viruses with which we are dealing. By definition, a virus that produces a chronic infection is one that has very little or no cytopathogenicity. That is, it must be able to infect a cell but not kill it or interfere severely with its metabolic processes . If the virus does kill the cell, or so inhibit the cell's metabolism so that it is badly injured, then the cell can't support the virus and the infection is terminated. If infection goes far enough to cause the host's death then the virus is without a home. Or turned the other way around, if the host musters a good immunologic defense to this kind of an injurious virus, the result would be an acute, short-lived infection, which would preclude chronic viral infection. So by definition, the viruses of chronic infection have very little cytopathogenicity.

There are three general kinds or groups of viruses that fall into this category. The first are the viruses that are really part of the host. The best example is the oncornaviruses. These are the RNA C type tumor viruses that have been isolated from virtually all birds and mammals with the possible exception of man. The current claims of such isolations from humans are still disputed, but if every other species has a C type virus, it will undoubtedly be demonstrated in man very soon. These viruses are such good symbionts that they have integrated themselves into the genome of the host that carries them. The murine oncornaviruses have been studied the most carefully, and every strain of mouse carries one or more of such viruses and has in its genome the information to make these viruses. Whether you chose to call the virus an exogenous agent or part of the host is a matter of semantics. But it's there. It has a characteristic morphology; you can separate it, put it into tissue culture and make it grow. This kind of virus is present then in any mouse one deals with. It is part of the animal and if it causes a disease, which it may well do, that disease is just part of the biology of the animal and cannot be eliminated. Many cancer workers believe this is true concerning the oncogenic potential of this virus. If there are such oncogenic viruses in man then they are part of man, and one has to deal with the cancer problem in man realizing that he may have in every one of his cells the potential to make a cancer producing virus.

The second class of virus is one that must be transmitted horizontally. It can come in the milk from the mother early in life or from another source later in life, but it is highly infectious and produces a chronic viral infection in almost all normal animals into which it is introduced. A good example is the Epstein-Barr virus in man. About ninety percent of the people in this room have antibodies to Epstein-Barr virus, which means that you were once infected with the virus and probably still carry it. Other examples are polyoma, a very common viral infection of humans, and Aleutian disease agent or virus, which infects almost all mink that are exposed to it. The strain of mink determines the severity of the Aleutian disease that follows, but the virus induces a life-long infection in most infected mink.

There is a third class, which ordinarily has the ability to cause an acute infection in naturally responding adult humans or animals. But in certain individuals this virus produces not acute infection, but chronic infection. This host doesn't make the usual effective immune response that causes fever and all the rest of things we associate with acute infection and elimination of virus, but instead covers up the viral agent and just holds it down without eliminating it. Ninety-nine percent of normal individuals who are exposed to measles get the usual acute disease--rash, fever, etc.-- and then recover. Occasionally, though, the host's immune response doesn't eradicate the virus, but puts enough antibody into the circulation so that those cells infected by measles choose to hide the evidence. They undergo modulation so the measles antigens that ordinarily would be on the surface of the cell are hidden inside. The host merrily goes on producing antibody, and cells that are infected keep their virus sequestered. The virus and the antibody don't meet, and the person doesn't have an acute infection. Probably much later, particularily if the virus is in the brain where apparently it can persist, the antigen is exposed and faces the antibody. Diseases such as SSPE can follow, often many years after the presumed initial contact. These then are the three kinds of viruses.

The host of the chronic viral infection by definition can't get rid of the virus or it wouldn't be a chronic infection, but on the other hand he is certainly not tolerant to the virus. There is no such thing as complete immunologic tolerance to any viral infection. Even to the oncornavirus infections, in which the viral genome is passed vertically with the germ cells of the parent, there is an immune response. In all of the species where this virus has been found, evidence exists that the host makes an immune response to the virus without eliminating it. And the disease that one subsequently sees is the product of that immune response against antigens from the virus or altered host-virus combinations. The more viral antigen and the more host immune reactants, the more severe the disease. With inbred mice one can pick out some strains that get very sick very early and others that live almost a normal life span and get a chronic disease very late as a result of infection with the same viral agent. This then gives you a picture of the kinds of disease that we are dealing with and the two principles, the receptive host and the noncytopathic virus, both of which are necessary for chronic immunologic disease to occur.

The first example I'd like to discuss is from the third class of virus, lymphocytic choriomeningitis (LCM). Although it infects both man and mice, only certain of these individuals develop chronic viral infection. Ordinarily, a normal adult mouse with a good immune response that is infected experimentally makes an immune response, eliminates the virus, and has excess antibody detectable. There is no evidence that the virus injures the cell directly, although there is an acute disease that clears up or kills the animal depending on how much virus is involved. If you put the same virus into a neonate via milk or by injection, or if you immunosuppress an adult so he can't make a complete immune response and then infect him, high levels of virus persist for the rest of these animals' lives. Until about ten years ago, it was suspected that neonatal exposure, when the immune system isn't well developed, would cause the animal to acquire tolerance. When he became immunologically mature, he found this virus present and accepted it as self. But, this theory isn't true. There is an immune response in this situation, and there is antibody that can be detected.

Mice chronically infected with LCM develop immune complex disease, particularly glomerulonephritis. Their glomeruli contain all the elements of immune complex disease--antibody or gamma globulin, complement and viral antigen. There are many such examples of glomerular deposits of complexes with identifiable viral or bacterial antigens in man.

In these LCM infected mice, we should find the complexes not only in the kidneys but also in the circulation , and in fact we were able to show that their sera were infectious. The next question was, how much of this infectious material is in complex form bound to gamma globulin or complement? The answer is, nearly all of it. After you remove the mouse gamma globulin with antibody to it, 2.5 logs of the LCM infectivity are lost. So, more than 99% of the total viral material in the circulation is stuck to gamma globulin, almost certainly in the form of antigen-antibody complexes. If you eliminate complement with anti-complement antibody almost the same kind of drop in infectivity follows; therefore, virus in the circulation is combined not only with gamma globulin but also with complement. To show that this is not an artifact or nonspecific precipitation of virus, one can take rabbit antiserum against mouse albumin and get a much bigger precipitation, of course, because there is more albumin in the circulation than gamma globulin or complement. But spinning down the albumin precipitate causes no change in the infectivity of the supernate, so the precipitation of the viral antigen with gamma globulin and complement appears to be specific. This clear-cut result and the fluorescent microscope picture that accompanies it are the first two bits of evidence that chronic viral infections induced at or before birth do not produce complete immunologic tolerance.

In addition to the fact that the infected animals form antibody, as you would guess, their lymphocytes become sensitized. Therefore, we asked the question, would splenocytes from sensitized or carrier mice kill cultured cells that were infected with LCM and were exposing LCM antigen on their surfaces? The targets were chromium labeled LCM infected embryo cells that were cultured with splenocytes from infected and control adult mice and examined at 6 hours and 18 hours for chromium release. With spleen cells from an uninfected animal there is a relatively small background of killing at 6 hours and not much more at 18 hours; but if one adds splenocytes from an infected animal, there is significant killing at 6 hours and over half the target cells are killed at 18 hours indicating that the splenocytes are sensitized and that these splenocytes or lymphocytes should have all the expected potential of killing infected cells within the body of the host.

This process is not limited to LCM viral infection. Biopsies of human glomerulonephritic kidneys have shown viruses in the glomeruli, e.g., hepatitis B, measles, Epstein-Barr, dengue and influenza viruses (Table 1). In animals the list of such virus induced immune complex diseases is much longer (Table II).

Now let's take an immunologic disease that occurs spontaneously in animals and see if we can find any evidence that viruses are involved. A good example is the rapidly moving, lupus erythematosus-like disease that begins at around 5 months of age in New Zealand black x New Zealand white hybrid mice and is fatal at around 9 to 11 months for females and at 15 to 20 months for males. In females at about 5 months of age anti-nuclear antibody begins to form, a month or two later proteinuria develops and two-three months later they die. Immunologically this disease is almost identical to systemic lupus erythematosus in humans, particularly in reference to the kinds of antibodies and the nature of the renal lesion. The early renal lesion of this immune complex glomerulonephritis is rich in polymorphonuclear leukocytes, and deposition of PAS positive material is evident in the glomerular capillary walls. If one uses immunofluorescent techniques to examine a kidney section for host gamma globulin, for complement, for DNA, which we know is one of the antigens

TABLE I

VIRUS INDUCED IMMUNE COMPLEX DISEASE IN MAN

1. Hepatitis B Disease (Australian Antigen)
2. Subacute Sclerosing Panencephalitis (Measles)
3. Infectious Mononucleosis
4. Dengue Hemorrhagic Fever
5. Burkitt's Lymphoma (EBV)
6. Influenza

TABLE II

VIRUS INDUCED IMMUNE COMPLEX DISEASE IN ANIMALS

1. Lymphocytic Choriomeningitis
2. Lactic Dehydrogenase
3. Murine Leukemia
4. Murine Sarcoma
5. Gross Leukemia
6. Friend Leukemia
7. Rauscher Leukemia
8. Rowson-Parr
9. Polyoma
10. Coxsackie B
11. Aleutian Disease of Mink
12. Equine Infectious Anemia
13. Hog Cholera

involved, or for one or more oncornavirus antigens, one sees their granular deposition in glomerular mesangia and capillary walls.

To find out what really is going on, one has to turn to a quantitative determination of immunologic events. The best we can do in this situation is to homogenize these kidneys and, at an acid pH, dissociate the immune complexes and elute the gamma globulin or antibody. Then we can ask, to what antigen has this antibody been formed? When we absorb this elute gamma globulin with insoluble nuclear protein that should react with most of the anti-nuclear antibodies, almost half of the gamma globulin eluted from the kidney is bound. So at least this much of it is anti-nuclear antibody. In addition, a significant amount, about 18%, reacts with the oncornavirus. These New Zealand hybrids, like all other mice, carry oncornaviruses so there is no reason why they shouldn't have been exposed to oncornavirus antigens. And just to show that these weren't the same antibodies absorbed by two different antigens, when we did both absorptions simultaneously, we accounted for about two-thirds of the antibody.

There are several lessons to be learned from these results. We know that the nuclear protein material we used contains a number of antigens to which the animal is making antibody. We know that there are at least a half dozen nuclear antigens to which the human lupus patient responds. We know now that in the oncornavirus there are six or seven specific antigens, and we know that the New Zealand hybrid mouse makes antibody to every one of these antigens. So two-thirds of the gamma globulin in these murine lupus kidneys reacts with at least 12 different antigens. Undoubtedly there are other antigens that we don't know about and can't identify until we suspect their presence and test for them. The point I would like to make is that these spontaneous diseases of both animals and man are not the result of a single antigen-antibody reaction, and it's not likely that the manipulation of a single antibody response will provide effective treatment.

Experimentally, in an animal genetically programmed to produce anti-nuclear antibody and anti-viral antibody, to develop spontaneous disease with multiple antigen-antibody systems, and to die at 9-11 months, what happens if there is an incidental chronic viral infection? Is the spontaneous disease affected at all? The answer is yes. To test this, we used either polyoma, a DNA virus, which when given to young mice doesn't hurt them other than to establish chronic infection or LCM virus, a RNA virus which in most murine strains causes little harm within the first 9 months of life. If New Zealand hybrids are given polyoma at or near birth, the appearance of anti-nuclear antibody in each mouse is greater. In New Zealand white mice, which are not normally subject to death from immunologic disease but live a normal life span, neonatal polyoma infection increases the incidence of anti-nuclear antibody. Furthermore, incidental chronic viral infection not only can cause viral-antiviral complex disease but also can trigger latent autoimmune responses in susceptible hosts. If you analyze the gamma globulin or antibody from the kidneys of these LCM infected animals, half reacts with nuclear protein antigens and an additional 28% reacts with LCM antigens. In comparison, SWR, an immunologically normal mouse, given the same amount of LCM at birth makes no antibody to nuclear antigens, but has a strong antibody response to the LCM antigen and an associated LCM-anti-LCM immune complex nephritis. It appears that an incidental viral infection doesn't make an animal do something that he is not gentically programmed to do, but rather hastens or magnifies his genetically determined responsiveness.

We said that in the spontaneous murine lupus, oncornaviruses seem to play some role. If all normal mice contain one or more oncornavirus usually expressed at low levels, what would the immunopathologic effect be of superinfecting these animals with oncornavirus? We began our work on superinfection by isolating a virus from the New Zealand mouse, since we wanted an isolate from animals with the disease that we were interested in. As it turned out this wasn't important. The virus we got from lymphoblasts of the New Zealand mouse, Scripps leukemia virus (SLV), is very much like Moloney virus. We infected immunologically normal hybrids, for example BALB/c x New Zeland mice, with varying doses of SLV and observed serum p 30, a measure of viral production, antinuclear antibody, lymphoma increased because this is an oncogenic virus. The amount of p 30 measured by radioimmunosassay increased as you expect, indicating the amount of virus formed. The incidence of anti-nuclear antibody rapidly reached near maximum as the animals responsed to this added horizontal oncornavirus infection. The incidence of glomerulonephritis increased with an increasing viral dose, and the incidence would be even greater except that many of the animals died of lymphoma before they had time to develop a demonstrable glomerulonephritis. Therefore, in an immunologically normal hybrid, one can get both anti-nuclear antibody and glomerulonephritis as a result of the super-infection with oncornavirus. Next, we induced similar SLV infections in a number of murine strains and observed that different strains of mice make different amounts of virus. It is important to note that the New Zealand black x white hybrid that gets lupus spontaneously makes very little virus. In other words, it has an ability to hold viral production down. What may be surprising is that this New Zealand hybrid mouse gets very little lymphoma. You could say that this animal then is more or less successfully handling the oncogenic challenge of the virus, although he does it at a price. The price he pays is a fatal immunologic disease, that is, high levels of anti-nuclear antibody and an almost uniformly fatal glomerulonephritis. It seems likely that this animal which suppresses, perhaps by immunological means, a viral infection and associated malignancy may in fact be doing so at the risk of developing an immunologic disease. This situation has implications for any vaccination programs that might be proposed if and when viral isolates from human tumors are developed. Would widespread prophylactic immunization against a ubiquitous virus of man, even if 100% protective against certain cancers, be desirable if it involved the risk of inducing a significant amount of immunologic disease? This is a very real consideration that would have to be tested carefully in reasonably large private studies and carefully controlled clinical studies.

In summary, first, one can say that viruses which cause chronic viral infections are certainly potent inducers of immunologic disease. Second, however, the immune responses involved are probably determined by the genetics of the host and therefore the character of the disease is determined by the genetics of the host much more than by the precise nature of the virus. This isn't a one virus-one specific disease situation. The predisposed individual's immune mechanisms, which are genetically determined, are abnormal and respond aberrantly to a variety of stimuli including several viruses. Finally, probably not in man, nor certainly in the mouse, will there be only one etiologic agent viral or otherwise for each immunologic disease. Rather there are likely to be varied and multiple causes for single immunologic diseases, a situation now apparent in glomerulonephritis. Immune complex glomerulonephritis with a single pathogenic mechanism may have dozens of different causes. I think that will be true for lupus and some of the other immunologic diseases. It is likely that these diseases are characterized by unusual immunologic responses to relatively ordinary antigenic substances. Any search for the etiologic agents of these diseases ought to be planned with this possibility in mind.

TRANSPLANTATION IMMUNOLOGY

John S. Najarian, M.D. and Ronald M. Ferguson, M.D.
University of Minnesota, Department of Surgery
Minneapolis, Minnesota 55455

The idea of whole organ transplantation for the purpose of replacement of disabled organs appears to date back to ancient times. As early as the second centruy B.C. the Chinese surgeon Pien Chiao is reputed, by legend, to have operated painlessly and transplanted successfully the hearts of two patients. However apocryphal the above example, the concept of organ transplantation seems to have occupied even the minds of the ancients. It was however, not until the development of adequate vascular anastomoses by Carrel and Guthrie (1,2) that technically feasible organ transplantation of vascularized grafts could be accomplished. Despite technical success, however, the results of these early workers were discouraging. Successful transplantation awaited the definition of the histocompatibility barrier, its genetic control, and the immunobiologic mechanisms involved in graft rejection.

An important land mark was the demonstration that skin grafts between identical human twins were accepted, whereas those between genetically different persons were regularly rejected. With this as a starting point, Gibson and Medawar studied skin allografts in burn patients and analyzed experimentally the fate of skin allografts in rabbits (3,4). These classic studies were the first real definitions of the basic pathophysiology of allograft rejection and its immunologic principles. The studies of Medawar clearly defined the relationship between genetically determined biologic individuality and the rejection of allografts.

The MHC and Genetic Laws of Tissue Transplantation

In most species of vertebrates studied there exists a tightly linked gene complex on the segment of one chromosome which controls a variety of immunologic traits of an individual within a species. This gene complex is called the major histocompatibility locus (MHC) and is phenotypically expressed not directly as many classical traits are, but by the ability of the gene products of this region to evoke specific immune responses in a histoincompatible animal. Thus, the phenotypic expression is one of a potential immunologic response. The MHC in man, called (HLA), has been divided into four regions, A, B, C, and D on the basis of identifiable markers for each region. These markers are expressed on the cell surface of virtually every cell in an individual. The A, B, and C traits are defined serologically by reaction against specific antibodies and the D locus is defined by the ability of lymphocytes from one individual bearing one D specificity to stimulate blast transformation and proliferation of lymphocytes from a second, unrelated D, different individual, a so-called "mixed lymphocyte reaction". There are certain conceptual characterisitcs of MHC gene products that are important to the understanding of the genetic laws of transplantation. First, the phenotypic products of histocompatibility genes are potential histocompatible antigens whose phenotypic manifestations depend upon the immune response they illicit in a recipient. Secondly, histocompatibility antigens are inherited co-dominantly; thus each allele for each locus inherited from each parent is expressed equally in a given individual. Thirdly, dissimilarity at a single MHC locus is usually sufficient for the rejection of an allograft.

From these features of histocompatibility genes, the outcome between various genetic combinations of donor and recipient can be predicted. The rules governing the outcome of skin grafts between defined inbred mouse strains were originally formulated by Little and revised by Snell and Stimpfling (5). These are known as the 4 laws of tissue transplantation. The first law: Transplants exchanged between genetically identical individuals (isografts) are expected always to be accepted permanently. An example of this is the high rate of clinical success of kidney transplantation between identical twins. Second law: Transplants performed between two animals within the same species, but differing at one or more MHC locus (allografts) are not successful without immunosuppressive therapy. Third law: Grafts from either inbred parent strain to an Fl hybrid or combination of those two inbred strains succeed, while grafts in the reverse direction are regularly rejected in a non immunosuppressed host. This is shown graphically in Figure 1. Fourth law: Fl hybrids between two inbred strains of animals characteristically will accept any graft from any animal genetically identical to the parental strain or any F1 hybrid combination of the two parental strains. The following table demonstrates these concepts looking at only a single H locus with 2 alleles.

The principles of immunogenetics defined above in the four laws of transplantation are based on the assumption that MHC genes are expressed co-dominantly each evoking equally strong immune responses in a recipient. Furthermore, it must be emphasized that these laws were formulated using inbred mouse populations and are

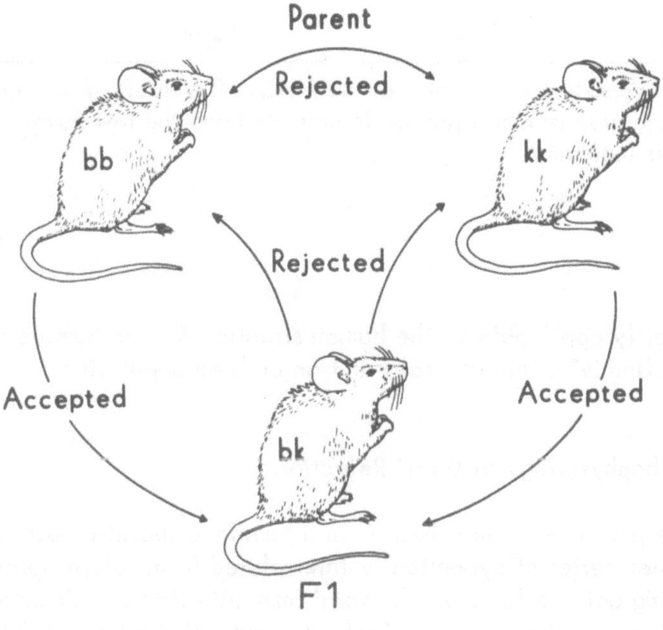

Figure 1: Genetic Control of Allograft Rejection in Inbred Mice.

Table I

Skin Graft Results Predicted by Genetic Laws of Transplantation

Donor	Recipient	Result	Law
xx	xx	take	(l)
	xy	take	(3)
	yy	rejection	(2)
xy	xx	rejection	(3)
	xy	take	(4)
	yy	rejection	(3)

x and y represent two alleles of the MHC. The result of skin grafting, i.e. rejection or non rejection is indicated and the law governing each result is indicated.

only partly applicable to the human situation for, in humans one is not dealing with inbred strains but an outbred population.

Pathophysiology of Graft Rejection

The presence of an allograft in a histoincompatible host sets off a complex series of dynamically interrelated immunologic processes involving both cellular and humoral immunity that are simultaneously occurring and directed specifically towards elimination of the graft bearing histoincompatible surface antigens. There are two phases of this allograft response. The afferent, or sensitization limb, whereby the host lymphoid system recognizes the graft as foreign and sets in motion that immunologic machinery necessary for getting immunocompetent cells "ready to act". Once sensitization has occurred there is an efferent or effector limb whereby the immunocompetent cells that have been sensitized "act" by specifically destroying the graft bearing the surface antigens to which the effector lymphoid cells have been sensitized.

Sensitization - the Afferent Limb

There are basically three mechanisms whereby a host becomes sensitized to a histoincompatible organ that has been transplanted. The most information in this subject available deals with renal allografts. The first involves soluble antigen. From the renal vein effluent of a transplanted renal allograft one can recover particulate antigen that can sensitize a second host to the antigens identical to those on the allograft and can bind specific antibody directed toward histocompatible antigens on the surface of the grafted organ. It is thought that this particulate antigen is shed by the graft into the circulation where it becomes trapped within lymph nodes. Once contained within the lymph node it is phagocytised by macrophages, processed and presented to lymphocytes, also contained within the lymph node, in a form which sensitizes these lymphocytes and confers on them the ability to recognize and destroy tissue bearing identical antigens. A second form of sensitization is the so called "passenger lymphocytes" contained within the allografted kidney. The highest concentration of histocompatible antigens of all tissues in the body are contained on lymphoid and hematopoetic cells. Therefore, lymphocytes are rich sources of cell bound antigens. These passenger lymphocytes can get into the host circulation and lymph nodes thus sensitizing the host, or host cells circulating through the transplanted graft can come in contact with these passenger lymphocytes and become sensitized. Thirdly, and probably the most significant form of sensitization, is the graft itself which naturally contains histocompatibility antigens on its cell surfaces. For example, within a kidney, uncommitted host lymphocytes circulate through the allograft coming in contact with its foreign antigens present on the surface of the allograft cells and from here either become sensitized within the graft or home back to lymph nodes or other lymphoid tissues and begin a maturation process whereby they become "ready to act". Of these three mechanisms of sensitization, shed particulate antigen, passenger lymphocytes and the allograft surface itself, the relative role of each and the degree of sensitization occuring by each mechanism described in a host is not known at present. It is generally thought however, that the allograft itself provides the bulk and most significant contribution to sensitization.

Allograft Destruction: The Efferent Limb

The immune response to an allograft is generally thought to be a cell mediated process resembling delayed hypersensitivity. Several observations have led to this conclusion. First, specific sensitivity to an allograft in mice can be transferred to a syngeneic animal by immune cells but not by immune serum, thus demonstrating the cell mediated nature of the response. Secondly, cell mediated responses are almost exclusively T cell mediated, and congenitally athymic or "nude" mice display indefinite survival of allografts as well as xenografts presumably because of the lack of the cellular machinery to mount an allograft response. Thirdly, T lymphocytes from animals bearing allografts have the capability in vitro of direct cell mediated killing of tissues bearing antigens identical to the sensitizing allograft.

Although the concept of rejection of allografts by cytotoxic T cells is of undoubted importance in allograft rejection, the recent discovery and assay ability in vitro of other cells that are imporant in transplantation immunity has led to several other proposed mechanisms for the destruction of allografts. The involvement of B cells in the production of allograft antibody, K cells in antibody dependent cell mediated killing as well as macrophage killing, all provide possible mechanisms capable of destroying allografts. In addition, immunoregulatory cells such as suppressor T cells and the role they play in the adaptation of an allograft must also be considered.

The following is a brief description of several proposed mechanisms of allograft destruction.

Cytotoxic T lymphocytes: Lymphocytoxicity mediated by

T lymphocytes has been demonstrated after the injection of allogeneic spleen cells, or after skin or tumor allografting in mice. The kinetics of cytotoxic cell generation after skin grafting show a peak correlating exactly with the time of rejection, suggesting an important role for these aggressor cells in the rejection process. However, it is interesting to note that when the allograft recipient is submitted to various treatments such as allogeneic antisera (6) or cyclophosphamide (7) one observes a disassociation between allograft rejection and the appearance of cytotoxic lymphocytes. For example, treatment of animals with donor specific allogeneic antisera prior to graft rejection only slightly delays the rejection of the allograft, but rejection occurs far before the appearance of cytotoxic T lymphocytes. Thus, other mechanisms either occuring concomitantly or in some time sequence relative to the development of cytotoxic T lymphocytes must be important in mounting a destructive allograft response.

B cells in antigraft antibody: It has been pointed out previously in this symposium that most immune responses are dependent on the interaction of various lymphocyte subpopulations. For example, antibody is made by plasma cells. These plasma cells are derived from B lymphocytes which in the presence of antigen, macrophages and other T cells are stimulated to differentiate into plasma cells which are then capable of secreting a class of antibody that shows specificity for the stimulating antigen. The T cell involvement in this instance is of a helper nature in that antibody cannot be produced or B cell differentiation stimulated in the absence of T lymphocytes. In the allograft response, antibody directed towards histocompatibility antigens on the graft is produced in a recipient. The kinetics of this antibody production closely resemble those of the development of cytotoxic T lymphocytes. Under these circumstances, antibody could bind to the allograft forming antigen-antibody surface complexes which can activate the complement system leading to direct membrane damage to the graft and subsequent recruitment of nonspecific effector cells such as polymorphonuclear leukocytes and/or macrophages to be attracted to the area of the allograft and themselves nonspecifically participate in the destruction of the graft.

K cells and ADCC: Recently, a mechanism of graft destruction involving both cellular and humoral components of the immune response has been described in vitro (8). This mechanism has been termed antibody dependent cell mediated cytotoxicity, or ADCC. Under these circumstances a special class of antibody is produced in minute quantities that does not fix complement but is capable of binding specific antigens on the surface of an allograft. Once antibody coated, the graft becomes the target of a population of unsensitized lymphoid cells that are capable of binding to the antibody coating the allograft target. A combination of allograft, antibody and the "K" cells is lethal to that target. Antibody alone or K cells alone do not cause cellular destruction. Thus, both non - complement fixing antibody, called lymphocyte dependent antibody in this circumstance and the effector "K" cell are required to produce destruction of the allograft.

Macrophage mediated killing: Macrophages are found in large proportions among the cells infiltrating human renal allografts undergoing rejection. The role of macrophages in cell mediated immunity has been the subject of a great deal of recent investigation (9). It is clearly established that resistance to infection with intracellular parasites involves a two step mechanism whereby immune T cells, when confronted with a specific antigen can elaborate various factors that activate macrophages. As a consequence of this activation, macrophages acquire an increased nonspecific macrophagocidal activity (10). The concept of macrophages being the effector cells of cell mediated immunity has been extended to a variety of immune reactions including allograft rejection. Recently, substantial evidence of the role of macrophages in in vitro cytotoxicity has been provided by the finding that normal macrophage could be made specifically cytotoxic by contact with allogeneically immune lymphoid cells or cell free supernates from cultures of such immune lymphoid cells (11). It has been suggested that immune T cells elaborate a specific factor which is cytophilic for macrophages and upon binding can specifically arm those macrophages to become cytotoxic. Thus, specific macrophage arming mediated by sensitized T lymphocytes could also provide an excellent mechanism for allograft destruction.

Although all of the above mechanisms undoubtedly contribute to the rejection response, the exact contribution of each to allograft destruction is not currently known.

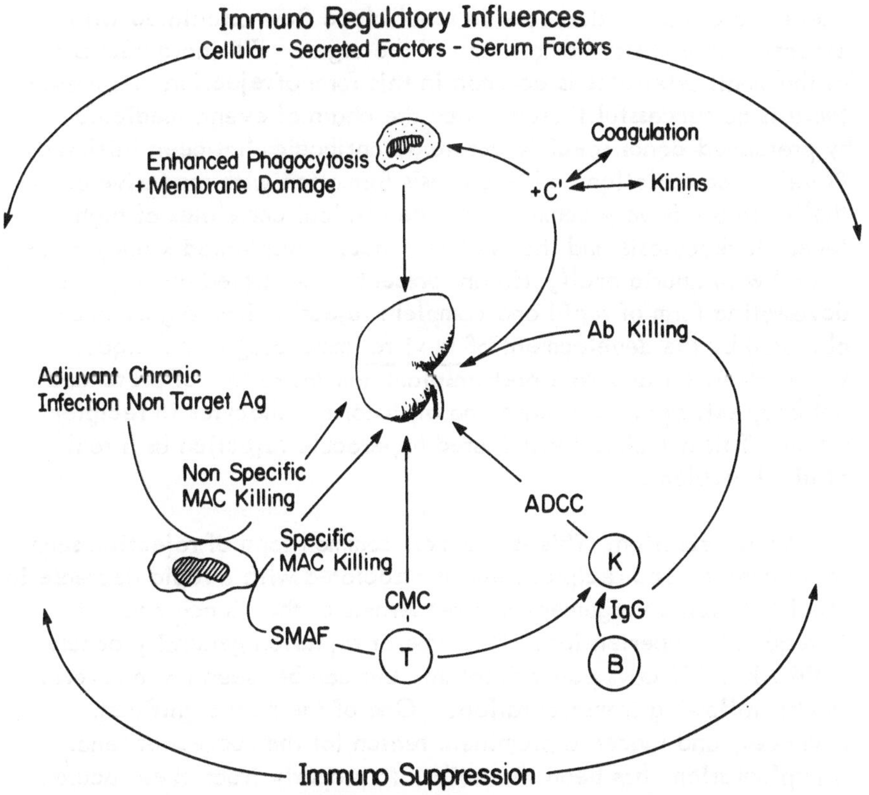

Figure 2: Effector Mechanisms of Allograft Rejection.

Types of allograft rejection: There are basically three types of immunologic rejection. Each of these has a characteristic time of appearance and light microscopic morphology. In addition, the immunologic mechanisms mediating each type of rejection are probably somewhat different. The examples of each given below are taken from human clinical renal allograft rejection.

Hyperacute rejection: This type of allograft rejection occurs within minutes to hours following transplantation and is associated with preformed antibodies of the cytotoxic type and directed specifically towards donor alloantigens. It is this type of immediate graft destruction that is screened for pretransplant by the cross-match technique utilizing recipient serum and donor lymphoid cells. Using this technique, the presence in a recipient of preformed cytotoxic antibody directed towards the donor is thus determined and clinical hyperacute rejection avoided. At operation, a transplanted kidney undergoing hyperacute rejection becomes swollen, blue and mottled.

There is a profound decrease in renal blood flow associated with extensive interstitial hemorrhage of the organ. Fibrinoid necrosis of the small arterioles is common in this form ofrejection. At present, there is no successful therapy once the chain of events mediated by preformed donor specific cytotoxic antibodies has been initiated. Platelet accumulation and thrombosis formation with extensive endothelial injury is very common and the clinical correlates of high fever, leukocytosis and the swollen tender transplanted kidney associated with anuria oroliguria are present. As stated above, this devastating form of rapid and complete rejection has largely been obviated by the development of in vitro immunologic techniques which allow for accurate pretransplant demonstration of preformed antibody utilizing cross matching of donor lymphocytes in recipient serum. This has almost eliminated hyperacute rejection as a real clinical problem.

Acute rejection: This is the most common form of rejection seen in an unsensitized recipient and is associated with a rapid decrease in renal function,enlargement and tenderness of the kidney, and not infrequently hypertension. This type of rejection generally occurs within 30 to 90 days post transplant, but can be seen up to several months following transplantation. One of the most significant advances, and indeed a prominent reason for the success of renal transplantation, has been the ability to properly treat these acute "rejection crises". Histologically, within the kidney there is evidence of acute mononuclear cell inflammatory response with perivascular accumulation of large immature mononuclear cells in the interstitium. The vasculature of the kidney is much less effected in acute rejection than it is in hyperacute rejection. There are large blast-like lymphoid cells present within the kidney and probably represent specifically sensitized cytotoxic T lymphocytes. The ability to immunologically detect acute rejection episodes prior to the development of renal damage and elevation of creatinine has not successfully been developed. It must be reemphasized, however, that even though significant renal damage has taken place during acute rejection episodes, such damage is largely reversible and successfully treated in a majority of incidents.

Chronic rejection: This type of rejection is seen during the course of most unsuccessful human renal allografts which fail months to years after good immediate post transplant function. It is characterized by slowly progressive renal failure and frequently hypertension. Histologically, there are findings of endothelial proliferation in small arteries and thickening of the glomerular basement membrane with eventual hyalinization, interstial fibrosis, chronic mononuclear cell infiltration and marked impairment of functional renal parameters. Unfortunately, unlike acute rejection episodes, chronic rejection is not responsive to therapy for the fibrotic component is not reversible.

Each of these types of rejection emphasizes a different immunologic mechanism. In the case of hyperacute rejection a totally humorally-mediated rejection reaction has been mounted. In this instance, antibodies bind to the endothelial cells in the small capillaries of the kidney and thus activate the complement sequence as well as the clotting cascade, thus leading to intravascular thrombosis of the small capillaries contained within the kidney and complement mediated membrane destruction of the graft. In the case of acute allograft rejection the response is almost totally cell mediated. In this instance, specifically sensitized T cells can be isolated from the graft which have the capability of killing in vitro target cells bearing donor alloantigens (12). During acute rejection episodes, cytotoxic antibody is most often not present and is only variably detected by immunofluorescent techniques on sections of a biopsied rejecting kidney. Chronic rejection on the other hand, probably involves a combination of both humoral and cellular responses. It has been reported that the appearance in a long term functioning renal allograft recipient of lymphocyte dependent antibody, or antibody that can mediate ADCC as describe above, correlates well with the ultimate appearance of chronic rejection. It could well be that the primary mode of immunologic graft destruction in this case is a slowly developing antibody dependent cell mediated destructive process.

Allograft Prolongation - Immunosuppression and Host Adaptation

It is now almost universally accepted that the combination of azathioprine and prednisone immunosuppressive therapy used together can effectively prolong renal allografts. The initial, rather emperical, observation made in man during the early days of clinical renal transplantation, established the effectiveness of this nonspecific kind of immunosuppression (13). This combination of drug therapy today is an essential feature of every clinical transplant center. The exact mechanism of immunosuppression induced by these drugs and any synergistic effect of the two drugs in combination, have been difficult to define. The clinical experience, however, is convincing and impressive. There has been little progress or change in the type of immunosuppression given transplant patients over the past twelve years. One notable exception is the use of antilymphocyte globulin (ALG) in conjunction with azathioprine and prednisone. It has been clearly demonstrated at the University of Minnesota (14) as well as other institutions, that ALG provides increased functional graft survival when combined with the standard azathioprine and prednisone therapy.

Immunologic Adaptation

It seems highly likely that in a recipient receiving nonspecific immunosuppressive therapy there may be certain "adaptations" occurring within the host's immune system in response to the organ allograft which renders that host less capable of mounting the specific destructive process involved in graft rejection. Whether such adaptation results in a reduction of the immunogenicity of the graft by alteration of the histocompatibility antigen present on the graft or whether it involves induction within the host of an immunoregulatory balance directed more toward acceptance than rejection of the graft is at present unknown. It is interesting in this regard to speculate on the role that the recently described suppressor cells may play in the whole process of immunologic adaptation to an allograft. There is little or no evidence that suppressor cells are active in such a process, but is an intriguing hypothesis and one that could conceivably be tested.

REFERENCES

1. Carrell, A.: La technique operatoire das airastomoses vasiulaires et al transplantation des visceres. Lyon Med. 99: 859, 1902.

2. Guthrie, C.C.: Applications of blood vessel surgery. Blood Vessel Surgery Lengman's, Green and Co.: New York, 1912, page 113.

3. Medawar, P.B.: J. Anat. 78: 176, 1944.

4. Gibson, T, and Medawar P.B.: J. Anat. (LInden) 77: 299, 1943.

5. Snell, G.O., and Stimpfling, J.H.: Biology of the Laboratory Mouse (Gwen, E.L. ed), New York, 1966, page 457.

6. Debray-Sachs, M., Soucy, P.E., and Hamburger, J. H. : J. Transpl. 110: 661, 1973.

7. Husberg, B.S.: Clin. Exp. Immunol. 10: 697, 1972.

8. Pearlman, P. and Holm, G.: Adv. Immunol. 11:117, 1969.

9. Unanue, E.R.: Adv. Immunol. 15: 95, 1972.

10. Evans, R., Cox, H., and Alexander, P.: Proc. Soc. Exp. Biol. 143: 256, 1973.

11. Dimitriu, A., Dy, M., and Hambruger, J.C.: J. Transpl. Proc. 7: 255, 1975.

12. Tilney, N.C., Strom, T.B., MacPhersen, S.G., and Carpenter, C.B.: Transplantation 20: 323, 1975.

13. Starzl, T., Marchioro, C., and Wadded, W.R.: Surg., Gynec. and Obstet. 117: 385, 1963.

14. Najarian, J.S., Simmons, R.L., Condie, R.M., et. al.: Ann. Surg. 184: 352, 1976.

TUMOR IMMUNOLOGY AND IMMUNOTHERAPY

Richard L. Simmons, M.D., Ronald M. Ferguson, M.D., Jon R. Schmidtke, Ph.D.

Departments of Surgery and Microbiology

University of Minnesota, Mpls., MN 55455

The first clear evidence that syngeneic tumors in experimental animals could be specifically recognized by the immune system of the host were studies in which inbred strains of mice were immunized by inoculation with syngeneic tumors. Using inbred animals with identical genetic background, the complicating factors of immunity against normal transplant antigens was avoided and specific reactivity against the tumor was assumed to be against antigens present on the tumor that were not present on normal tissues of the host.

Most tumors, both in humans and experimental animals, have antigens on the cell surface of tumor cells that are capable of inducing an immune response in their hosts (1). This has been demonstrated by several experiments. If in an animal bearing a syngeneic tumor, that tumor is totally removed or otherwise destroyed, lymph node cells or spleen cells from such an animal are capable of conferring, on a genetically identical animal, resistance to that particular, but not other, tumors (2). Likewise, the same lymph node cells from an "immune" animal are capable of killing tumor cells in culture (3). Immunotherapy seeks to take advantage of the antigenic character specific for each tumor by either altering the tumor to increase its antigenicity or by increasing the host's immune response to an unaltered tumor, or a combination of both.

Prior to considering the various types of tumor immunotherapy a few words about the immunologic environment in which tumors arise is appropriate. If an animal develops an autochthonous tumor, and that tumor is allowed to grow, there is an early concomitant immunity to the tumor but this wanes and a nonspecific kind of immunosuppression ensues with increasing tumor size and tumor bearing period. It is within the context of this altered and immunosuppressed environment that tumor immunotherapy must act. In brief "once established, a tumor and a host act synergistically and favoring the growth of the tumor" (4). Immunotherapy of cancer seeks to reverse this trend by altering those elements of the immune response to favor tumor cell destruction rather than its growth.

It is theoretically feasible to augment an immune response to a tumor in several ways. Each of these theoretical considerations has been translated into an experimental model in animals of tumor immunotherapy and some have been applied to human tumors. A general discussion of each of the model systems and its human implication follows.

Nonspecific active stimulation. This form of immunotherapy seeks to nonspecifically activate the host's immune apparatus with adjuvant substances such as BCG or *Corynebacterium parvum*. Both substances derived from bacteria, are known to increase nonspecifically the immune responsiveness of an animal. For example, adjuvant substances are capable of stimulating the appearance of copious amounts of antibody in response to antigens compared to the responses evoked without concomitant adminstration of adjuvants. The earliest experiments using such an approach to the treatment of malignancies were described by Coley who used a crude bacterial toxin extract to treat advanced malignancy (5). Additional support for this concept in humans derived from the observation that patients with lung carcinoma who developed emphyzema demonstrated increased survival over those patients who had courses that were uncomplicated by infection (6). Of all the immunoadjuvants that have been studied both in experimental animals and in humans, by far the most promising is the adjuvant derived from bacillis Calmette-Guerin (BCG strain of *Mycobacterium bovis*). Studies in mice have shown that BCG can be used to protect animals from the growth of spontaneous tumors or tumors induced by viral and chemical carcinogens (7). The most promising form of administration of the adjuvant in tumor immunotherapy is by intratumor inoculation. Administration of BCG in this fashion seems to effect two mechanisms, local tumor necrosis and the induction of systemic immunity to the tumor. These may well be independent mechanisms of the same or even differing cell populations in the inflammatory mixture that infiltrates the tumor as a result of BCG therapy.

Adoptive immunotherapy. The fact that tumor rejection is mediated largely by lymphoid cells and that animals bearing tumors lose both specific anti-tumor as well as generalized immune competence during tumor growth has prompted attempts to adoptively transfer immunocompetent lymphoid cells directed against the tumor as a method of immunotherapy against cancer. Several approaches to adoptive immunotherapy have been taken. One deals with the transfer of syngeneic cells from one animal immune to a tumor to a syngeneic animal bearing the tumor. Another approach, but probably less promising, involves the use of immunocompetent cells allogeneic, or non-identical, to the tumor bearing animal. Each of these adoptive immunotherapeutic approaches can be combined with other cancer anti-cancer modalities, and each alone has its own defined limiitations and restrictions in terms of practical potential for man.

It has been convincingly demonstrated that lymphoid cells taken from an animal immune to a tumor can transfer tumor immunity to an animal genetically identical to the tumor immune animal (8). The problem with this kind of approach is that such syngeneic in vivo sensitizations are impossible in man. However, an interesting study designed to determine whether tumor metastases could be prevented by immunotherapy was performed by Treves et al (9). A lung carcinoma was implanted in the foot pad of mice, and the local tumors were removed seven days after inoculation. Almost all of the mice died of lung metastases within 4 to 6 weeks. If however, one day following the tumor excision mice were treated with syngeneic lymphocytes from spleens that had been sensitized in culture against the tumor cells, a drastic reduction in the number of metastases and an increased survival of the treated animals was observed. Thus, once a solid tumor mass has been removed there are apparent metastic foci, not yet discernable by histologic means, which can be destroyed by specifically in vitro sensitized syngeneic lymphocytes. In addition, this model obviates the need for in vivo sensitization in syngeneic donors.

Although a promising model in experimental animals the use of *in vitro* sensitized syngeneic lymphocytes adoptively transferable for the treatment of human tumors has been attempted with little success (10). The problem here is generating in culture large enough numbers of specifically sensitized anti-tumor cells.

Specific active immunotherapy. This concept derives from the fact that tumor antigens are generally poor immunogens capable of eliciting only a low degree of immune responsiveness. It is possible, however, to increase the immunogenicity of tumor antigens and thus supplement the ineffective immunity in a tumor bearing host by increasing or even breaking the unresponsive state of the animal. Antigens can be rendered more immunogenic by altering the dose, physical state or the route of administration of a sensitizing tumor vaccine. Of all the techniques used to alter the surface antigenic character of tumors, only *Vibrio cholerae* neuraminidase (VCN), an enzyme that cleaves sialic acid residues from cell surfaces, has proven to be of value in the immunotherapy of established cancer. VCN has been shown to be capable of increasing the immunogenicity of a variety of strong and weak transplantation antigens both *in vivo* and *in vitro* (11, 12). On the basis of this Simmons et al (13) demonstrated that small, but firmly established methylcholanthrene-induced fibrosarcomas in mice could be made to regress by inoculation of tumor bearing mice with tumor cells having been treated previously *in vitro* with VCN. The effect could not be induced with cells treated with heat inactivated VCN. The regression was immunospecific and could be induced only with VCN treated cells identical to the type growing in the host. The successful treatment of other syngeneic and allogeneic tumors has also been demonstrated using a vaccine of VCN treated tumor cells. In murine leukemia systems tumor regression induced by VCN treated leukemia cells has been obtained (14, 15).

The regression of established spontaneous mammary tumors was induced by combination of active specific immunotherapy using a VCN treated tumor cell vaccine in combination with nonspecific active immunotherapy using injections intratumor of BCG (16). Immunotherapeutic models utilizing VCN tumor vaccines have been combined with other anti-tumor modalities. For example, the combination of chemotherapy and immunotherapy with VCN treated cells has been found to be antagonistic in some systems, a finding which might be expected since most chemotherapeutic agents are immunosuppressive. However, the proper use of chemotherapy to reduce a tumor mass and of immunotherapy to "mop up" surviving tumor cells as a concept is a strong theoretical possibility and indeed has been shown to be possible (17) using a spontaneously occuring lymphoma in mice.

Passive transfer of informational substances. Another form of adoptive transfer immunotherapy which attempts to bypass problems involved with adoptive transfer of whole cell preparations utilizes the passive transfer of subcellular components from a sensitized population of lymphocytes to confer a state of immunity in a secondary host. The most promising of the informational substances is so-called "immune RNA". RNA is extracted from spleen cells of animals bearing a specific tumor,and these in turn are incubated with normal non-immune syngeneic spleen cells. The syngeneic recipients of the RNA treated spleen cells were found to be resistant to the growth of a sarcoma isograft. These results have been repeatedly confirmed. There is also good evidence that the passively transferred immunity is a property of immune RNA. Non-immune RNA is ineffective, and RNA-ase, an enzyme which breaks down RNA, destroys the activity of the specific transfer of immunity (18).

In addition to the protection from subsequent challenge with a tumor (or immunoprophylaxis) recent studies have demonstrated complete tumor specific regression of established guinea pig hepatoma tumors by a combination of therapy utilizing 1) xenogeneic immune RNA extracted from immune animals, 2) unsensitized syngeneic peritoneal exudate cells, and 3) immunization with tumor specific antigen preparations. This combination of adoptive transfer and active specific immunization for tumor immunotherapy conferred on the tumor bearing animals a systemic immune response strong enough to destroy small but established tumors (19).

Other forms of immunotherapy have been attempted but were less successful. These include possible administration of anti-tumor antibodies directed towards tumor specific antigens (20) or the administration of anti-tumor antibodies conjugated with toxic substances such as diphtheria toxin or a cytotoxic drug (21). This concept involves the homing and concentration of a toxic substance in the area of a tumor by conjugating that toxic substance to an antibody that will selectively bind to the tumor. The use of such an immunotherapy model has been attempted in humans with cutaneous melanoma with limited early success (22).

Although successful tumor immunotherapy can be achieved in experimental animals and preliminary studies with human cancers seem to indicate that there is a possible role for immunotherapy in the treatment of human tumors, one must consider the place of immunotherapy in the context of other available therapeutic modalities. Immunotherapy as a primary means of treatment for human tumors is highly unlikely. However, it has been repeatedly shown in experimental models that with a limited tumor load immunotherapy can be advantageous. Thus, a form of adjuvant immunotherapy that can complement such well established primary treatment modalities as surgery, radiotherapy or even chemotherapy, shows great potential. However, at the present time our understanding of how a normal host immune response, both cellular and humoral, is altered in response to an autochthonously growing spontaneously arising tumor and how, at various stages of tumor growth the degree of antigenic load or tumor size affects the host's immune response are presently poorly understood. Until a greater understanding of the degree and changing character of the host's immune response to his tumor is elicited, effective human immunotherapeutic protocols will probably not be of great use. However, the recent explosion of knowledge in the field of immunology, coupled with the intense research efforts being directed towards tumor immunology suggest that in the future immunotherapy as an adjuvant treatment may be very useful.

REFERENCES

1. Hellstrom, K.E., and Hellstrom, I.: Adv. Cancer Res. 12: 167, 1969.

2. Smith, R.T.: New Engl. J. Med. 278: 1207, 1968.

3. Hellstrom, I., and Hellstrom, K.E.: Int. J. Cancer 4: 587, 1969.

4. Smith, R.T.: New Engl. J. Med. 278: 1207, 1968.

5. Yashphe, D.J.: In Immunological Parameters of Host-Tumor Relationships (D.W. Weiss, ed.), Academic Press, New York, 1971, p. 90.

6. Ruckdeschel, J.C., Codish, S.D., Stranahan, A., and McKneally, McKneally, M.F.: New Engl. J. Med. 287: 1013, 1972.

7. Baldwin, R.W., and Pimm, M.W.: Conference on the Use of BCG in Therapy of Cancer, National Cancer Institute Monograph, No. 39, 1973, p. 11.

8. Old, L. J., Boyse, E.A., Clarke, D.A., and Carswell, E.A.: Ann. N.Y. Acad. Sci. 101: 80, 1962.

9. Treves, A., Cohen, I., and Feldman, M: J. Natl. Cancer Inst. 54: 777, 1975.

10. McKhann, C.F.: in Transplantation (J.S. Najarian, and R.L. Simmons, eds.)., Lea and Febiger, Philadephia, 1972, p. 297.

11. Simmons, R.L., Lipschultz, M.L., Rios, A., and Ray, P.K.: Nature: 231: 111, 1971.

12. Simmons, R.L., Rios, A., Ray, P.K.: Nature 231: 179, 1971.

13. Simmons, R.L., Rios, A., Lundgren, G., Ray, P.K., McKhann, C.F., and Haywood, G.R.: Surgery 70: 38, 1971.

14. Bekesi, J.G., Arneault, G., and Walter, L.: J. Natl. Cancer Inst. 49: 107, 1972.

15. Kollmorgen, G.M., Erwin, D.N., and Killion, J.J.: Proc. Amer. Assoc. Cancer Res. 14: 69, 1973.

16. Simmons, R.L., and Rios, A.: Surgery 71: 556, 1972.

17. Bekesi, J.G., and Holland, J.F.: Rec. Results in Cancer Res. 47: 357, 1974.

18. Pilch, Y. Veltman, I., and Kern, D.: Surgery 76: 23, 1974.

19. Paque, R.E., Meltzer, M., Zbar, B., Rapp, H., and Dray, S.: Cancer Res. 33: 3165, 1973.

20. Smith, R.T.: New Eng. J. Med. 287: 439, 1972.

21. Ghose, T., Cerini, M., Carter, M., and Nairn, R.: Brit. Med. J. 1: 90, 1967.

22. Oon, C.J., Apsey, M., Buckleton, K.B., Cooke, I., Hanham, I., Hazarika, P., Hobbs, J., and McLeod, B.: Behring Inst. Mitt. 56: 352, 1974.

IMMUNE DEFICIENCY AND MALIGNANCY

John H. Kersey, M.D.

Dept. Lab. Med. & Pathol. and Dept. Pediatrics

University of Minnesota, Minneapolis, MN 55455

Accumulating evidence suggests than an understanding of the immune system will assist in the analysis of malignant adaptation. A large body of evidence indicates that patients with malignancies of various types also have immunologic deficiency which may involve both the cell-mediated and humoral systems. The types of malignancy with demonstrable immune deficiency include l) epithelial malignancies, e.g., those involving breast, stomach, colon, and other sites; 2) nervous system tumors of varying types; and 3) a variety of mesenchymal tumors including sarcomas. In many instances the degree of immune deficiency correlates with the extent of the malignancy, suggesting that much of the immune deficiency in cancer patients is secondary to the cancer (1). The causes of this secondary immune deficiency in cancer patients are undoubtedly several and probably include nutritional factors and production of immunosuppressive proteins (e.g., alpha fetoprotein) by the tumor (2,3). Because of this secondary immune deficiency, it is currently not possible in most cancer patients to determine what role, if any, immune deficiency plays in causing the tumor. However, the purpose of this presentation is not to discuss secondary immune deficiencies, but rather to concentrate on primary immunodeficiencies in order to determine the possible role of immune deficiency in the development of malignancies in humans. This analysis is made possible because of three relatively well defined immune deficient populations: The first consists of patients with primary, genetically-determined immunodeficiency; the second is composed of patients undergoing renal transplantation who receive long-term immunosuppression; and the third involves ageing humans, i.e., those in the "golden years."

An analysis of patients with genetically-determined immunodeficiency includes study of a variety of immune deficiency syndromes, most of which affect children (4). Shown in Table 1 are incidence rates and estimated risk values for each of five syndromes: 1) congenital (X-linked) immune deficiency, a disease involving a defect in B lymphocytes; 2) severe combined immunodeficiency which involves both T and B cells; 3) isolated IgM deficiency; 4) Wiskott-Aldrich syndrome, a disease involving abnormalities of T cells, B cells and macrophages; and 5) ataxia-telangiectasia which involves cutaneous blood vessels and the nervous system as well as being associated with abnormalities of T and B cell function (5). Common variable immune deficiency is generally late in onset, and frequently results in abnormalities of both cell-mediated and humoral immunity. Extensive analysis of the possible association between immune deficiency and cancer was begun through establishment of an Immunodeficiency-Cancer Registry at the University of Minnesota. Correspondence with physicians caring for these patients indicated that approximately 2800 patients were at risk for development of malignancy during the last 20-25 years. All patient groups developed severe infections and most patients died of infections of varying types. About 7% developed and died of malignancy in this analysis in 1964. This represents a significantly increased risk over the general populations, most of which are children. Comparison with the age-match populations revealed that the risk is about 200 times that of the general population (6).

Our next analysis concerned the type of malignancy which these immune deficient patients develop, and the results were quite striking. It was evident that most malignancies were lymphoid or lymphoreticular in origin. Details are presented in Table 2. Of the total, 57% were solid lymphoreticular malignancies, 27% were leukemias, 20% were epithelial, 2% mesenchymal, and 4% were malignancies of the nervous system. Some differences were noted between the various types of immune deficiency although the numbers are too small to be significant.

The second group of patients with immune deficiency and malignancy are comprised of the renal transplant recipients. Renal

Table I

Evidence of Malignancy in

Primary Immunodeficiency Syndromes*

Disease	Incidence	Estimated Risk
Congenital X-linked immunodeficiency	6/approx. 100 9/approx. 400	6%
Severe Combined system immunodeficiency	9/approx. 400	2%
IgM deficiency	6/approx. 70	8%
Wiskott-Aldrich syndrome	24/approx. 300	8%
Ataxia-telangiectasia	52/approx. 500	10%
Common variable immunodeficiency	41/approx. 500	8%
Total	138/approx.1870	7%

*From Kersey, J. et al.: Int. J. Cancer 12: 333, 1973

Table II

Immunodeficiency-Cancer Registry; Summary of Cases

Primary Immunodeficiency Disease	Histologic Type: Lymphoreticular %	#	Leukemia %	#	Epithelial %	#	Mesenchymal %	#	Nervous System %	#	Total Cases
IgA Deficiency	31	4	·	·	54	7	7.5	1	7.5	1	13
X-linked (Bruton's) Agammaglobulinemia	33	4	58	7	·	·	·	·	8	1	12
Variable Immunodeficiency	47.6	28	5	4	43	24	1.7	1	1.7	1	57
Severe Combined Immunodeficiency	55	6	45	5	·	·	·	·	·	·	11
Ataxia-telangiectasia	60	42	23	16	13	9	1	1	3	2	70
IgM Deficiency	71	5	·	·	14	1	·	·	14	1	7
Wiskott-Aldrich Syndrome	84	28	6.5	2	·	·	3	1	6.5	3	34
TOTAL	57	117	17	34	20	41	2	4	4	9	205

transplant recipients who receive suppressive drugs are also at an increased risk for development of malignancy. Most of the malignancies are lymphoreticular as with congenitally immunodeficient patients. These data have been analyzed extensively by McKhann, Penn, and others (7,8). Details presented by Hoover and Fraumeni indicate that the risk ratios of lymphomas in males and females are 32 and 38, respectively (9). This predominance of reticulum cell sarcomas is also seen in the analysis of the congenital immunodeficiency syndromes (Table 3). Most lymphomas which develop in genetic and drug-induced immunodeficiency appear in younger individuals. However, ageing individuals also have immune deficiency, and therefore are likely at a high risk of development of lymphoid malignancies. Details are presented in Figure I. Further evaluation of the cause of these lymphoid malignancies may be better understood by delineation of the cellular origin of the malignancy (i.e., whether there is origin in T cells, B cells, or monocytes). Surface marker analysis is currently available to detect T lymphocytes, B lymphocytes, and monocytes by use of specific markers (Table 4).

Surface marker methods have recently been applied to lymphoid malignancies from a wide variety of lymphoid malignancies generally without known predisposing immunodeficiency. A number of laboratories, including ours, have analyzed malignant lymphoid cells for surface markers. Results from these analyses indicated age differences. Childhood lymphomas, for example, generally have origin in T lymphocytes, while adult lymphomas generally have origin in B lymphocytes. Chronic lymphatic leukemia, a disease of adults, is a B cell disease. Acute lymphatic leukemias in childhood frequently have origin in T cells, but less frequently are of T cell origin in adults. It has been shown that while children have a higher proportion of T cell malignancies, there is a striking increase in B cell maligancies with age.

The suggestion that there is a link between B cells, malignancy, ageing, and immunodeficiency makes the prediction that B cell malignancies should predominate in persons with congenital or drug-induced immunodeficiency. There is some evidence to support this notion. First, a number of "reticulum cell sarcomas" have been shown to have origin in B lymphocytes (10), Gajl-Peczalska, K. and

Table III

Lymphoreticular Malignancies by Cell Type Reported in 117 Individuals with Seven Primary Immunodeficiency Diseases.*

Year of Cancer Diagnosis, 1949-1975

Tumor Type Reported	Number of Cases
reticulum cell sarcoma	22
lymphosarcoma	21
lymphoma, Not Otherwise Specified (NOS)	18
Hodgkin's disease	18
malignant reticuloendotheliosis	8
malignant lymphoma	7
lymphoreticular, NOS	5
undifferentiated lymphoma	2
lymphoblastic lymphosarcoma	2
reticular lymphosarcoma lympho-epithelial thymoma malignant reticulosis small cell lymphosarcoma generalized reticuloendotheliosis reticulum cell lymphoma malignant lymphosarcoma histocytosarcoma undifferentiated round cell sarcoma malignant lymphogranulomatosis histocytosis reticulosis thymoma with lymphocytic lymphoma Burkitt's lymphoma histiocytic lymphoma	1 each (15)

*Collected by the Immunodeficiency-Cancer Registry, 1972-1975.

Table IV

Markers of Human Peripheral Blood Mononuclear Cells

	B Cells	T Cells	Multiple Marker Lymphocytes	Monocytes
Surface Ig	+	-	+	-
Human B lymphocyte antigen (HBLA)	+	-	?	-
Sheep erythrocyte receptors (E rosette)	-	+	+	-
Human T lymphocyte antigen (HTLA)	-	+	?	-
Fc receptors (aggregated IgG or EA rosette)	+	-	+	+
Complement receptors (EAC rosette)	+	-	+	+

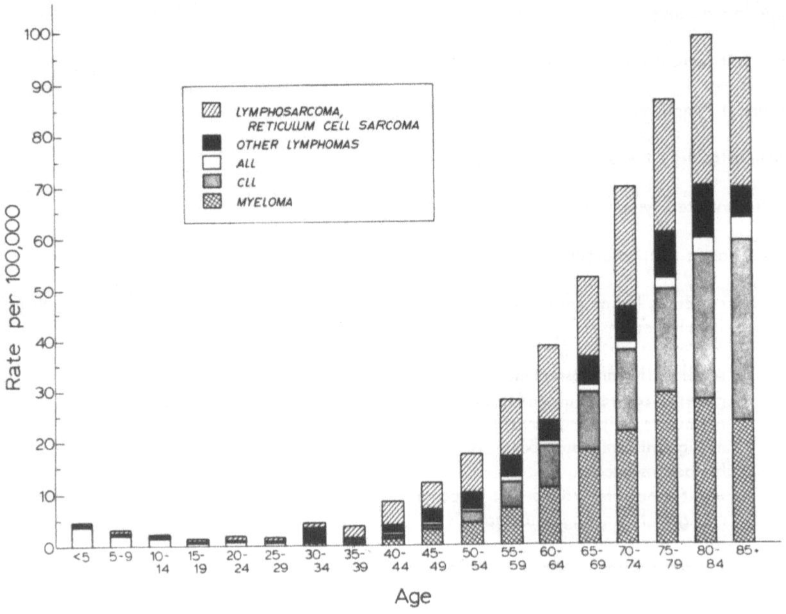

Figure I

Age Related Incidence of Malignancy

Kersey, J., (unpublished observations). Histopathologic examination also provides support. Some malignancies which develop in immunodeficient patients clearly are of B cell origin when examined morphologically, as in the Minnesota case in which the brain was involved. To date, few lymphoid malignancies in genetic or drug induced immunodeficiency have been analyzed using surface markers. However, two children with primary immunodeficiency syndromes are known to have developed B cell malignancies. One of these is a case of ataxia-telangiectasia in which a B cell malignancy developed (C. Nezelov, personal communication). The other is a case from Toronto in which a child with severe combined system immunodeficiency developed a polyclonal proliferation of B cells with gammopathy (II).

The relationship between immunodeficiency and lymphoid malignancy is complex and may reflect a variety of pathogenetic mechanisms. Some are summarized in Table 5. A favorite speculation of mine links immune deficiency, genetic defects, ageing, and lymphoid malignancy. The basic speculation, as shown in Figure 2,

Table V

POSSIBLE MECHANISMS RESPONSIBLE FOR INCREASED RISK OF LYMPHORETICULAR MALIGNANCY IN PERSONS WITH IMMUNODEFICIENCY

1. Deficiency of cellular regulatory mechanisms (eg., deficiency of suppressor cells).

2. Chronic antigenic stimulation with viruses, fungi, bacteria, alloantigens resulting in enhanced cellular proliferation.

3. Increased malignant transformation due to chromosomal abnormalities (eg., ataxia-talangiectasia).

4. Infection with exogenous oncogenic viruses resulting in enhanced malignant transformation.

5. Deficiency of humoral regulatory mechanisms, eg. antibody.

6. Activation of endogenous oncogenic viruses.

7. Defective immunologic destruction of malignant lymphoreticular cells (modified immunologic surveillance hypothesis).

Figure 2

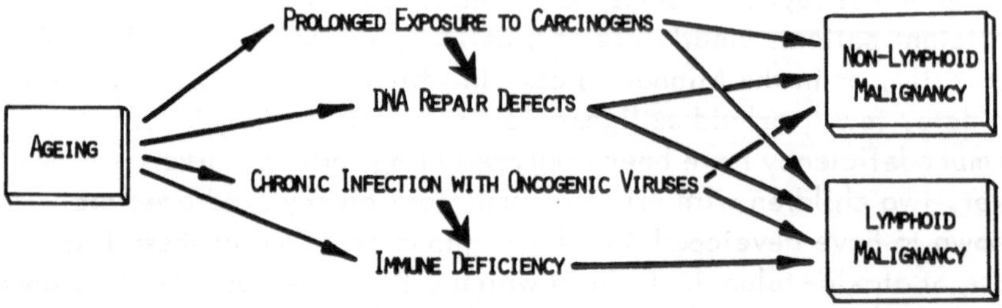

suggests that ageing is central in malignant adaptation. Central to pathogenesis of both lymphoid and non-lymphoid malignancies are prolonged exposure to carcinogens, DNA repair defects, and chronic stimulation with oncogenic viruses. Immune deficiency is suggested to be central to the pathogenesis of lymphoid malignancy, but not nonlymphoid malignancy.

In summary, persons with immune deficiency associated with genetic defect, drug-induced immunodeficiency associated with renal transplantation, and ageing appear to be at greatly increased risk of development of lymphoid malignancy, especially of the B cell type. Future study should provide characterization of the various factors responsible for this malignant adaptation.

REFERENCES

1. Fleisher, T.A., and Kersey, J.H.: Immunologic mechanisms in the prevention and therapy of cancer. Am. J. Dis. Child. 128: 739, 1974.

2. Murgita, T.A., and Tomasi, T.B.: Suppression of the immune response by a-fetoprotein. J. Exp. Med. 141: 440, 1975.

3. Purtillo, D., Kersey, J.H., Hallgren, H., and Yunis, E.: Alpha fetoprotein: Clinical use and biologic implications. Am. J. Clin. Path. 59: 295, 1973.

4. Good, R.A., Biggar, W.D., and Park, B.: Immunodeficiency in man. In: Progress in Immunology, B. Amos, ed., Academic Press, N.Y., 1971, p. 700.

5. Kersey, J.H., and Spector, B.D.: Immune deficiency diseases. In: Persons at High Risk of Cancer: An Approach to Cancer Etiology and Control, Academic Press, Inc., N.Y., 1975, p. 55.

6. Kersey, J., Spector, B.D., and Good, R.A.: Cancer in children with primary immunodeficiency disorders. J. Pediatrics 84: 263, 1974.

7. McKhann, C.F.: Primary malignancy in patients undergoing immunosuppression for renal transplantation. Transplantation 8: 209, 1969.

8. Penn, I., and Starzel, T.: Immunosuppression and cancer. Proc. 4th Congress Transpl. Soc. Abstracts 220, 1972.

9. Hoover, R., and Fraumeni, J.F., Jr.: Risk of cancer in renal transplant recipients. Lancet 2: 55, 1973.

10. Brouet, J.C., Preud'homme, J.L., Flandrin, G., Chelloul, N., and Seligmann, M.: Membrane markers in histiocytic lymphomas (reticulum cell sarcomas). J. Nat. Cancer Inst. 56: 621, 1976.

11. Gelfand, E.W., Baumal, R., Huber, J., Crookston, M.C., and Shumak, K.H.: Polyclonal gammopathy and lymphoproliferation after transfer factor in severe combined immunodeficiency disease. New Eng. J. Med. 289: 1385, 1973.

IMMUNOLOGICAL SURVEILLANCE OF CANCER

Robert S. Schwartz, M.D.
Hematology Service, Department of Medicine
Tufts University School of Medicine, Boston, Mass.

Tumor immunology can be divided into two broad aspects. One of these deals with the immunology of established neoplasms and has as one of its important goals the development of clinically effective immunotherapy. Almost the entire armamentarium of immunology has been applied to this problem. Signs of progress are evident, but much still needs to be learned.

The second major branch of tumor immunology deals with immunologic defenses against incipient tumors. The fundamental premise underlying this work may be summarized by the concept of immunological surveillance. Stated concisely, this theory contends that malignant cells elicit a protective immunological reaction by virtue of unique antigenic determinants on their surfaces. This reaction eliminates incipient neoplasms perhaps by the same type of immunological response that destroys grafts of foreign cells (1,2).

The idea of immunological surveillance has had a profound effect on tumor biology. Apart from its important theoretical implications for the pathogenesis of cancer, the theory makes a prediction that should concern many physicians. This is that spontaneous or iatrogenic immunosuppression will render an individual highly susceptible to the development of neoplasms. If, as the theory contends, mutant and potentially neoplastic cells arise within each of us frequently, then depression of the immune response should weaken the defense against these cells with a resulting increased risk of cancer. Since agents with immunosuppressive actions are widely used, the implications of immunological surveillance are highly relevant to clinical medicine. Although patients with spontaneous immunodeficiency diseases and immunosuppressed recipients of organ grafts are relatively unusual, thousands of patients with a variety of autoimmune disturbances undergo treatment with immunosuppressive drugs and tens of thousands of patients receive immunosuppressive anti-cancer agents. Therefore, we need to examine carefully the validity of this theory which, if substantiated will bring about important changes in clinical practice.

Elsewhere I have remarked that a major difficulty with the theory of immunological surveillance is that it has been inadequately tested (3). Stutman (4) has also discussed this situation, which is a curious anomaly because, as a general rule, scientists prefer to test the validity of a theory by designing experiments that will challenge it. The more resistant the theory is to refutation, the more acceptable it becomes (5). Einstein's theory of relativity is a classic example. Physicists have for decades devised challenges to relativity, yet it has withstood all of them. In so doing, its credibility has been vastly strengthened.

In the case of immunological surveillance, the reverse has been true. Instead of challenging the theory, investigators have designed experiments with the sole purpose of proving it. All too often the results of such experiments have been predictable and by and large, unworthy of the theory.

For example, it can be predicted that mice infected with virulent oncogenic viruses and treated with anti-thymocyte serum will develop high incidence of neoplasms (6). This is so because it is known that the principal immunological defense against infection by viruses originates in thymus dependent lymphocytes. There is no way these results distinguish between immunological defense against viruses and immunological surveillance against neoplasms. Yet, such experiments have been repeated again and again, always with the same erroneous conclusion.

Apart from this difficulty, little notice has been taken of important exceptions to the predictions to the theory of immunological surveillance. For example, the demonstration that neonatal thymectomy, a procedure that cripples the cellular immune system, actually decreases the incidence of mammary carcinomas in mice (7). Another exception not taken into account by the theory is the failure of neoplasms to develop in high incidence in immunologically privileged sites (3,4). Areas of the body such as the anterior chamber of the eye, the brain, subcutaneous fat pads, and the cheek pouch of the Syrian hamster are functionally isolated from the immunological system. They contain virtually no lymphocytes, and if allografts are implanted within them they are rejected only very slowly. The expectation of the theory is that such sites should be cancer "hot spots". They are not. Indeed, the incidence of cancer in these areas seems to be lower than in other sites with free access to lymphocytes (3,4).

Nude mice possess a gene that renders them hairless and deprived of a thymus. They have no cellular immunity because they lack thymus-dependent lymphocytes (8). According to the theory of immunological surveillance, these mice should have a high incidence of multiple neoplasms. This has not been the case (9). Outzen et al (10) have maintained a colony of nude mice under strict germ-free conditions, and thereby protected them against premature death by infection. As they aged, these mice did develop a high incidence of neoplasms, but the singular and very important finding was that virtually all of the tumors arose from the lymphoreticular system. The surveillance theory predicts that a great variety of tumors should arise in these athymic mice.

A similar situation applies to immunodeficient humans. For example, about 10% of patients with spontaneous immunodeficiency diseases develop neoplasms, a proportion much higher than in immunologically normal persons of the same age. As in the nude mice, over 80% of the tumors originated from the lymphoreticular system (11).

The same findings apply to renal transplant recipients, all of whom are treated with immunosuppressive drugs. The overall incidence of neoplasms in these patients is 200 times the anticipated rate (12). Yet, only two varieties of cancer are common -- those of the skin and malignant lymphomas. The incidence of reticulum cell sarcomas in women who received a renal transplant was 700 times the anticipated rate. Yet the incidence of the commonest neoplasm in women, breast cancer, was not increased (12).

Another aspect of malignant growth that seems incompatible with immunological surveillance is that it is almost always clonal in origin; that is, all the cells of a given neoplasm arise from a single ancestor (13). This has been demonstrated for virtually all lymphomas and for almost all carcinomas tested up to now. Burkitt's lymphoma is a striking example. This disease seems casually related to infection by the Epstein-Barr virus (14). This virus can infect all B cells, yet the tumor that arises is the descendant of only a single B cell (15). Since all B cells infected by this virus possess the same antigenic composition, it seems unlikely that a surveillance mechanism selectively eliminated all infected potentially malignant cells but one. Even if we accept this tenuous argument, it contains within it a contradictory seed: one cannot accept a theory that postulates a failure of immunity and simultaneously argue that neoplasms are the result of immunoselection (16).

In light of these and other problems with the theory of immunological surveillance, it seems reasonable to seek other explanations for the documented increased incidence of neoplasms in immunologically suppressed individuals. An example of alternative possibilities may be found in recent studies of patients with ataxia telangiectasia, a complex immunological deficiency disease associated with a high incidence of lymphoreticular neoplasms. Evidence of chromosome abnormalities that antedate the neoplasm has been uncovered (17). The skin fibroblasts from these patients are unusually radiosensitive and, a defect in the mechanism that repairs the defective DNA has been found (18, 19). These results present a valid alternative explanation to the extraordinary susceptibility of patients with ataxia telangiectasia to neoplasms.

Other studies suggest that immunosuppressive chemicals like cyclophosphamide and azathioprine may be mutagens (20,21). If they also produce cancer promoting mutations, this may explain why patients treated with them and similar agents could be prone to cancer.

Finally, we need to consider the possibility that defects in the regulation of lymphoproliferation promote lymphoid neoplasms. If lymphocytes proliferate in response to antigens under conditions of abnormal control, could this not lead to lymphoma (22)? Here we may be dealing with a system analogous to the development of endocrine gland tumors after a disruption of hormonal feedback loops (23).

The theory of immunological surveillance has been criticized in several recent reviews (3,4,11,16). The conclusion of these analyses was that, when examined in detail, the data failed to support the theory. A surveillance system may operate in certain restrictive situations, but it can no longer be accepted as a general explanation. Nevertheless, the theory has been of immense value because it forced us to consider new explanations for the pathogenesis of malignancy. And, in the final evaluation, the true measure of a theory is not whether it is right or wrong, but whether it leads to a new level of understanding.

REFERENCES

1. Burnet, F.M., 1970. The concept of immunological surveillance. Progr. Exp. Tumor Res. 13:1.

2. Klein, G., 1973. Tumor immunology. Transpl. Proc. 5: 31.

3. Schwartz, R.S., 1975. Another look at immunologic surveillance. New Engl. J. Med. 293: 181.

4. Stutman, O., 1975. Immunodepression and malignancy. Adv. Cancer Res. 22: 261.

5. Magee, B., 1973. "Karl Popper", Viking Press.

6. Hirsch, M.S., and Murphy, F.A., 1968. Effects of anti-thymocyte serum on Rauscher virus infection of mice. Nature 218: 478.

7. Martinez, C., 1964. Effect of early thymectomy on development of mammary tumors in mice. Nature 203: 1188.

8. Wortis, H.H., Nehlsen, S., and Owen, J. J., 1971. Abnormal development of the thymus in "nude" mice. J. Exp. Med. 134: 681, 1971.

9. Rygaard, J., 1973. "Thymus and Self". John Wiley and Sons, New York.

10. Outzen, H.C., Custer, R.P., Eaton, G.J., et. al., 1975. Spontaneous and induced tumor incidence in germfree "nude" mice. J. Reticuloendothelial Soc. 17:1.

11. Melief, C.J.M., and Schwartz, R.S., 1975. Immunocompetence and malignancy in "Cancer, a Comprehensive Treatise", Vol. 1 (F.F. Becker, Editor). Plenum Press, New York.

12. Hoover, R., and Fraumeni, J.F., Jr., 1973. Risk of cancer in renal transplant recipients. Lancet 2: 55.

13. Friedman, J.M., and Fialkow, P.J., 1976. Cell marker studies of human tumorigenesis. Transplant. Rev. 28:2.

14. Miller, G., 1974. The oncogenicity of Epstein-Barr virus. J. Infect. Dis. 130: 187.

15. Fialkow, P.J., Klein, E., Klein, G., et. al., 1973. Immunoglobulin and glucose-6-phosphate dehydrogenase as markers of cellular origin in Burkitt lymphoma. J. Exp. Med. 138: 89.

16. Moller, G., and Moller, E., 1976. The concept of immunological surveillance against neoplasia. Transplant. Rev. 28: 1.

17. Hecht, F., McCaw, B.K., and Koler, R.D., 1973. Ataxia telangiectasia-clonal growth of translocation lymphocytes. New. Engl. J. Med. 289: 286.

18. Taylor, A.M.R., Metcalfe, J.A., Oxford, J.M., and Harnden, D.G., 1976. Is chromatid-type damage in ataxia telangiectasia after irradiation at G_0 a consequence of defective repair? Nature 260: 441.

19. Paterson, M.C., Smith, B.P., Lohman, P.H.M., Anderson, A.K., and Fishman, L., 1976. Defective excision repair of γ -ray damaged DNA in human ataxia telangiectasia fibroblasts. Nature 260: 444.

20. McCann, J., and Ames, B.N., 1976. Detection of carcinogens as mutagens in the Salmonella/microsome test. Proc. Nat. Acad. Sci. 73: 950.

21. Byrnes, J.J., Downey, K.M., Black, V.L., and So, A.G., 1976. Azathioprine as a mutagen and carcinogen. J. Clin. Invest. 57: Abstract 461A.

22. Schwartz, R.S., 1972. Immunoregulàtion, oncogenic viruses, and malignant lymphomas. Lancet 1: 1266.

23. Furth, J., 1975. Hormones as etiological agents in neoplasia in "Cancer: A Comprehensive Treatise" Vol. 1 (F.F. Becker, Editor). Plenum Press, New York.

INDEX